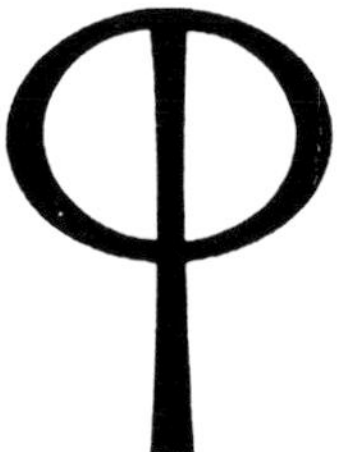

Jacobo Schifter, PhD

Public Sex in a Latin Society

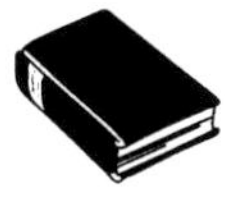

Pre-publication REVIEWS, COMMENTARIES, EVALUATIONS . . .

"This is another rich and challenging addition to the literature on sexual identity cultures and practices from the pen of Jacobo Schifter and his colleagues at ILPES. . . . This book combines an irresistible style and content with innovative theoretical insights that lay open the data and neatly extract new and challenging complexities surrounding the negotiation of sexual identities and desires. . . . As with all of Schifter's work, the presentation of findings that are vivid and arresting in their detail is accompanied by an insightful theoretical commentary. . . . *Public Sex in a Latin Society* rewards readers on two levels—it is both bewitching and evocative while remaining intellectually challenging. Having read it in one sitting, one is drawn back to an immediate second reading."

Gail Hawkes, PhD
Department of Sociology, Manchester Metropolitan University, Manchester, United Kingdom

More pre-publication
REVIEWS, COMMENTARIES, EVALUATIONS . . .

"***P****ublic Sex in a Latin Society* is an important book that contains rich information about the behaviors of men who have sex with men. Homosexual contact is a major transmission route for HIV in the Latin American region, but very little is known about the behaviors, mixing patterns, and attitudes of this population. This book is the most thorough exploration of this topic that I have seen. The information provided is crucial to the development of effective HIV/AIDS-prevention programs.

Jacobo Schifter and his colleagues at ILPES are to be commended for the thorough research they have conducted. It is a very readable book that rewards the reader with a wealth of knowledge and deepens our understanding of the attitudes and beliefs that form the behavior of these men."

John Stover
Vice President,
The Futures Group International,
Glastonbury, CT

The Haworth Hispanic/Latino Press
An Imprint of The Haworth Press, Inc.

NOTES FOR PROFESSIONAL LIBRARIANS AND LIBRARY USERS

This is an original book title published by The Haworth Hispanic/Latino Press, an imprint of The Haworth Press, Inc. Unless otherwise noted in specific chapters with attribution, materials in this book have not been previously published elsewhere in any format or language.

CONSERVATION AND PRESERVATION NOTES

All books published by The Haworth Press, Inc. and its imprints are printed on certified pH neutral, acid free book grade paper. This paper meets the minimum requirements of American National Standard for Information Sciences-Permanence of Paper for Printed Material, ANSI Z39.48-1984.

Public Sex in a Latin Society

THE HAWORTH HISPANIC/LATINO PRESS
Latin Sexuality
Jacobo Schifter, PhD, Senior Editor

Public Sex in a Latin Society by Jacobo Schifter

The Sexual Construction of Latino Youth: Implications for the Spread of HIV/AIDS by Jacobo Schifter and Johnny Madrigal

Public Sex in a Latin Society

Jacobo Schifter, PhD

The Haworth Hispanic/Latino Press
An Imprint of The Haworth Press, Inc.
New York • London • Oxford

Published by

The Haworth Hispanic/Latino Press, an imprint of The Haworth Press, Inc., 10 Alice Street, Binghamton, NY 13904-1580

Cover design by Jennifer M. Gaska.

Cover photo © Steven Underhill, www.steven-underhill.com

Library of Congress Cataloging-in-Publication Data

Schifter, Jacobo.
[Caperucita Roja y el lobo feroz. English]
Public sex in a Latin society / Jacobo Schifter.
p. cm.
Includes bibliographical references and index.
ISBN 1-56023-985-9 (hardcover : alk. paper).—ISBN 1-56023-986-7 (pbk. : alk. paper).
1. Homosexuality, Male—Costa Rica. 2. Gay men—Costa Rica—Sexual behavior. 3. Public spaces—Health aspects—Costa Rica. 4. AIDS (Disease)—Costa Rica. 5. Safe sex in AIDS prevention—Costa Rica. I. Title.
HQ76.2.C6713S353 1999
306.76′62′097286—dc21 99-16945
CIP

CONTENTS

ABOUT THE AUTHOR

Jacobo Schifter, PhD, is the Regional Director of ILPES (the Latin American Health and Prevention Institute), an AIDS-prevention program financed by the Netherlands' government. One of the most prolific writers in Latin America, Dr. Schifter wrote books on the Costa Rican civil war, U.S.-Costa Rican relations, and Costa Rican anti-Semitism before shifting his interests when AIDS started to affect the Central American region. He then established the first regional institute to fight the epidemic and created dozens of innovative programs, such as AIDS hotlines and AIDS-prevention workshops for Latin gays, prisoners, street children, Indians, male sex workers, and other minority groups. Dr. Schifter also started to publish controversial books on AIDS, including *The Formation of a Counterculture: AIDS and Homosexuality in Costa Rica* (1989), *Men Who Love Men* (1992), *Eyes That Do Not See: Psychiatry and Homophobia* (1997), *Lila's House* (1998), *From Toads to Queens* (Haworth, 1999), and *Macho Love* (Haworth, 1999). These books have become best-sellers in the region and have also played a part in changing many Latin governments' discriminatory policies against people with AIDS.

Preface

This book seeks to answer several key questions. What could have made a traditional gay Latin culture drastically change the rules of the game and take over public places to exhibit what was once forbidden? What factor or factors have triggered this change? Do these public places constitute a danger for the spread of HIV? How was Costa Rica's gay community able to reduce HIV infection and the numbers of gay men with AIDS? Is it possible for homosexuals to significantly change their desires and sexual practices? What are the typical public sex places in a Latin American setting, how do they work, and how do they evolve? Who are the main actors, and what are their motivations and their problems? How do the different groups that participate interact and influence one another and what are the main communication problems? Why are gay men murdered and how could these killings be prevented? Is public sex in a Latin country always "progressive"?

To answer these questions, the Research Department of ILPES began a qualitative and quantitative investigation in 1989 which has taken almost a decade. Our main mission, as always, was to investigate patterns of gay behavior in order to take effective prevention measures against HIV infection. It has never been our interest to denounce these activities nor to persecute those who practice them. On the contrary, we believe that public sex provides a number of opportunities that enable a sector of the population to "work through" certain problems of sexual communication and even to learn about safe sex. Therefore, we use fictitious names for people and places and have changed the locations and some of their characteristics to protect the people who have helped us so much in this investigation. We are also aware of the great dangers that lie in wait for participants and have thus paid considerable attention to them. In recent years, many gay men have been murdered by clients who frequent public sex places and we believe that our study can offer some basic safety rules.

One of ILPES' objectives is the empowerment of sexual minorities. We feel that these groups have not had much of a voice, and have been still less the subject of social research in Latin America. Although traditional studies usually quote their interviewees, the latter tend to remain under the dictates of the author, who provides us with the overall and final interpretations. In our case, we have tried to give a greater participation to our respondents, respecting their language and their way of seeing things, as well as giving them a voice in many of our analyses. We have found, for example, that criminals can analyze their own crimes better than we can, and also that active participants in public places can be excellent ethnographers. However, this way of "democratizing" a research project also has its problems. There were times when we would have wished that much of the data gathered were more "politically correct" and that the language used by these minorities were less coarse and rude to sensitive ears. We would also have preferred a less homophobic brand of humor from our interviewees, including the gays themselves. But we believe it is better to portray them as they really are, without the terrible censorship of their language that is so characteristic of Latin American social science.

This study was carried out by a team of professionals who are in the vanguard of research on sexual minorities. Among them are Rodrigo Vargas, a statistician and key organizer of this study; Dino Starcevic, a journalist; Luis Villalta, coordinator of the Listen to Your Voice project for former prison inmates, who carried out the research with the police officers; Antonio Bustamante, director of the El Salon program for juvenile delinquents in street gangs; Abelardo Araya, coordinator of the Movimiento 5 de Abril program for gays and lesbians who assisted in the ethnographic observation of public places; Lidia Montero, director of the ILPES publishing company; and Hector Elizondo, coordinator of the 2828 program for young street gays, who helped me contact many of the sex workers.

To all of them, my most sincere appreciation for their great work.

Despite the enormous debt I owe to all who participated in this study, the responsibility is mine alone.

Introduction

THE PORNOGRAPHY REVOLUTION

According to Michel Foucault, history has no predetermined course, nor is there any evidence to suggest that knowledge and experience are cumulative, or that changes take place as a result of scientific progress.[1] Instead, change is provoked by accidents and interruptions. In his analysis of the origins of the clinic, this philosopher and historian shows us how the plague and the concentration of corpses, rather than scientific discoveries, led doctors to begin carrying out autopsies. This fortuitous event was responsible for the shift from symptomatic medicine, in which disease was diagnosed on the basis of sight and hearing, toward modern medicine based on touching and internal examination.[2]

Along with Foucault, we believe that accidents and fortuitous events generate small revolutions in thinking. It is quite probable that if homosexual culture in Costa Rica—and possibly in Latin America in general—had not been confronted with a historic trauma, it might have remained hidden in the closet.

Costa Rica is a small country in Central America and one of the few nations in the world with an official religion. As in Iran, there is no separation between religion and the state. Thus, the public education system includes religious instruction for all students. All Costa Ricans contribute through their taxes to the salaries of senior clergymen. The Church is represented at all official government functions and there is no aspect of national life that is not influenced by it. On Christian feast days, the entire nation stops its activity to make way for celebrations. Until a few years ago, for Catholics, it was a crime to drive during Christian holidays. They would persecute those who were thought to disrespect them. Therefore, they would throw stones at vehicles that drove around during the holy days of Easter Week. The country is still so religious that government buildings are filled with religious images. Prayers are still said in public and private institutions. The majority of the country's villages are named after saints and God is even invoked in the televised weather forecasts. "Tomorrow, God willing, it will rain," says the weather reporter.

When a new government takes office, its first official act is to visit the Virgin of Los Angeles, the "national patron." Once a year, when the Virgin is flown by helicopter from her permanent home in Cartago to the capital, San José, the archbishops ask the faithful to take out small mirrors (to reflect the sunlight) to greet her as she passes over the rooftops of their homes. An article published by *La Nación,* Costa Rica's leading daily, reports that "this weekend, the Virgin will be in Talamanca," as if she were a living person.[3] Anyone who is not familiar with the customs of the Costa Rican people might conclude that the small stone statue had gone on vacation.

The Church has the power of veto in many public and private decisions. When a group of lesbians tried to organize a conference in the country in 1987, the Church protested to the government for having given permission to the organizers and stirring up public opinion against the event. In response, the then minister of security, who later became the president of Congress, declared that he would not allow the foreign participants to enter the country. The minister boasted that the lesbians would be easily recognized at the international airport. People made jokes about him, saying that this brilliant politician had invented a "lesbometer" to spot them.[4]

To date, the Costa Rican government has been unable to offer sex education in the nation's high schools. The Catholic Church rejected the instruction manuals that were prepared for this purpose, arguing that the texts contained "moral irregularities." The Church demanded changes to embrace its own vision of sexuality, which is opposed to premarital sex, nonreproductive sexual practices, abortions, most family planning methods, respect for sexual diversity, and condom use. The Church has also asked that the instruction manuals be imparted, among others, by those who are the least expert in the subject: priests.

It is hardly surprising that religious censorship promotes ignorance. For example, approximately 40 percent of young people are not sure or do not know whether a girl's first menstruation signals the start of her fertile period, and only 30 percent know when a woman is most likely to get pregnant. In addition, there are many myths: approximately 55 percent of young people of both sexes believe that masturbation is harmful and a slightly lower percentage believe there are vaccines to prevent sexually transmitted diseases.[5]

Costa Ricans traditionally conduct their sex lives by compartmentalizing them. In other words, in their heads they separate theory from practice. The Church's sexual discourse is not questioned, but, in heterosexual relations, people do otherwise than the Church tells them. This pattern is similar to what the *criollos* (Spaniards born in the New World) did during the colonial era with respect to the laws of the mother country: "I obey, but I don't comply," in other words, "I don't question authority, but I do what I like."

In the New World, slavery, the subordination of the indigenous people, and the need for cheap labor made it impossible to uphold Christian rules that allowed sex *only* within marriage. Costa Rica's poverty during the colonial period and its remoteness from the seat of political power, which for centuries was based in Guatemala, made for a poorer Catholic Church with fewer resources to impose its vision of sexuality.[6]

The Catholic Church preached chastity before marriage and prohibited adultery and divorce. However, it also had to coexist with a population exposed to undermining forces. The shortage of workers during the colonial period and the country's incorporation into international markets through coffee exports in the nineteenth century created a great demand for labor and for migrant populations, which in turn encouraged acceptance of children born out of wedlock.

Faced with a different economic and political reality, people opted to disregard many religious principles. Catholic writers admit that in spiritual matters Costa Ricans were more concerned with form than with content. The Catholic Church had to adapt itself to the reality that "conversion was never total." With respect to the Hispanic population, Blanco notes that the Christian faith was assimilated more by form than by intellect.[7]

To profess the Catholic faith and not obey its moral dictates has been characteristic of the Costa Rican people and of Latins in general: 42 percent of all births take place outside of marriage; men have an average of ten more sexual partners than women; 18 percent of babies are born to mothers under the age of twenty; 45 percent of pregnancies are unwanted;[8] the annual divorce rate is 20 percent; 35 percent of all women endure physical or psychological aggression from their partners; 27 percent of university students have been victims of sexual abuse as children,[9] and every year, nearly 5,000 abortions are induced.[10]

In Costa Rica, the people with scant education and those from the lower social and economic groups are the ones who, on average, have the highest birth rates. Whereas the fertility rate among the middle classes is 3.01, among the lower classes it is 4.17, or 30 percent higher.[11] It is precisely this sector of the population that is most religious and is most affected by the Church's anti-family planning policies.[12] For the middle and upper classes of society, when family planning measures fail, there is always the possibility of having an abortion in Miami.

However, for the Catholic Church to fight the infidelity of the majority of the population is like swimming against the tide. Its response has been to close its eyes to the "moral failings" of Costa Ricans and of its own priests, some of whom have recognized their own children publicly.

If there is a double standard in heterosexual relations, it is not hard to imagine the situation with regard to homosexuality.

In this sphere, people also say one thing and do another, though in a very different context. During the 1950s, for example, the police would raid gay bars and shave the heads of clients so that they would be recognized in the street. These practices continued without formal resistance until 1987.

Up until the mid-1980s, the attitude of Costa Rican gays was no different from that of heterosexuals: the dominant Catholic discourse on sexuality was not questioned, nor was it followed to the letter. Costa Rican gays, along with their fellow homosexuals in the rest of Latin America, learned to live a double life in which hiding one's homosexuality was as important as practicing it. Although there was never an explicit agreement between the state, the Church, and homosexuals, certain rules of coexistence or minimum tolerance levels were established:

1. It was forbidden to question the prevailing religious discourse and the lack of respect for minority rights, as well as the normality and morality of heterosexuality.
2. Gay sex was to remain totally hidden from the public. The issue of homosexuality was banned in the press, in sexual education, and in artistic productions.
3. A small number of gay bars were allowed to operate, only to prevent homosexuals from meeting in the streets, but there would be no official recognition of their activities. Much less would there be acceptance of public gay venues such as restaurants, leisure centers, hotels, and other places. The few bars that were tolerated had to pay bribes to remain open.
4. It was forbidden to establish public gay organizations.
5. The Church could attack homosexuals in a different way from heterosexuals. Unlike the latter, homosexuals were a small minority who could be blamed for all of the country's moral woes.

These rules—which were never made official but were faithfully obeyed—meant that the lives of Costa Rica's gay men were deeply closeted. Clients of gay bars lived in fear of being arrested, owners had to pay bribes to be allowed to stay open, and middle-class gays did most of their socializing at private parties. To be revealed as gay meant social disgrace and financial ruin, while being in the closet offered a certain privacy and other benefits. In a survey carried out in 1989, we found that many Costa Rican gays lived in deep hiding. When asked who knew of their sexual orientation, 55 percent of those who frequented bars admitted that their fathers did not know, and 40 percent of mothers were also unaware of their orientation, along with 49 percent of their doctors and 68 percent of their neighbors.[13]

Life in the closet caused problems but it also had its benefits:

1. Given that the issue of homosexuality as a lifestyle was censored, the media portrayed it as a criminal act. To the heterosexual public, being a homosexual was equivalent to being a thief, a satyr, or a murderer.
2. Given this image of sexual orientation, there was no benefit for gays in revealing their identity. On the contrary, being

exposed as a homosexual meant dismissal from one's job and rejection by one's family. The price to be paid for revealing homosexuality was social death.

3. This distorted image actually helped homosexuals: people had trouble recognizing gays because they associated them with criminals and could not conceive that an ordinary person might be gay. Thus, few homosexuals were persecuted and the majority passed unnoticed. They could live together, travel, and socialize with other men without others suspecting that they were couples. Moreover, Latin machismo, a culture that excludes women, actually worked in their favor: both heterosexual and homosexual men tended to socialize more with each other than with women, as Carrier also discovered in Mexico.[14]

Foucault does not believe that changes in thinking occur as a result of an accumulation of experiences or scientific developments. This is shown in the fact that the Stonewall riot (the gay protest in New York) in 1969, the upsurge of the gay movement in the United States, the debate among psychiatrists on homosexuality, and the struggle for peace in Central America did not change the status quo for gays in Costa Rica. Although Oscar Arias, Costa Rica's president from 1986 to 1990, received the Nobel Peace Prize for his mediation efforts in the Central American armed conflict, his government carried out the worst raids against the country's gay bars. So long as the price of revealing one's sexual identity remained high (in other words, the repression was overwhelming) and the closet offered certain benefits (the possibility of certain reduced spaces for homosexuality), the gay population showed no sign of questioning the status quo.

George Simmel believes that oppressed groups who opt to "accommodate" or adapt themselves to a disadvantageous situation always get less than they hope for.[15] This "accommodation" may last years, centuries, or millennia, but it is a fragile arrangement. The subordinate sectors have accepted a less than ideal situation and will always be alert to any attempt by the dominant groups to alter the terms of the arrangement. They will also seize any opportunity to improve the disadvantageous situation in which they find themselves, either when their power increases or when their subordination becomes intolerable. All situations of subordination are, according to Simmel, prerevolutionary. At a certain moment, any spark can light the fire.

In Costa Rica there was no Vietnam War or liberation movement for blacks and women to trigger a U.S.-style "Stonewall."[16] Thus, although the North American gay movement had some influence in the country, things essentially remained the same during the decade of the 1970s and part of the 1980s. However, by the mid-1980s, the situation was to change radically. The closet would no longer be a safe place and homosexuality would become visible in two ways: through political organization (which is not the subject of this book) and the upsurge in public sex.

AIDS AS A TRIGGER

In the case of Costa Rica, information about AIDS arrived before the first cases appeared in 1983. Despite this, the epidemic spread quickly. Given their homophobic attitudes, the authorities thought that so long as the disease claimed only homosexual victims, why try to stop it? The reactions of hostility, panic, repugnance, hate, and rejection that gays with AIDS suffered in hospitals made homosexual oppression more evident than ever before. Stories of nurses—both male and female—who refused to go near patients, doctors who made fun of their mannerisms, and microbiologists who refused to perform blood tests on homosexual patients clearly showed that the situation was intolerable. The Catholic Church's persecution was no less virulent. It used the epidemic to blame sexual "immorality" as the cause:

> AIDS is . . . a warning. There is a divine plan, a certain order; if men do not follow this, there are signs that show us things are going badly. We already knew that the problem of AIDS was coming: it is written in the Bible, but people do not know it; they ignore it. In a world like ours, full of evil and destruction, men kill each other, there are vices, homosexuality. . . . That is why AIDS has appeared.[17]

But the epidemic had another impact more threatening than social hostility: the end of anonymity. Soon the Ministry of Health began tracing the sexual partners of those who were infected with the supposed intention of asking them to take an HIV test. Since AIDS patients were required to supply the names of all their sexual partners in the past ten years, soon half of the gay community was on these lists. In a small country such as Costa Rica, where there is neither confidentiality nor anonymity, the majority of active homosexuals were at the mercy of a homophobic health minister.

The HIV test itself became a source of "outing." The fact that several people were involved in the process of tracing contacts, interviewing, taking blood samples, and testing and recording results made it impossible to guarantee confidentiality. For many gay men, the mere fact of being summoned for an interview on suspicion of HIV infection was a way of being dragged out of anonymity. The heterosexual population began to realize that the image it had of homosexuals was false, and it lost its "innocence" with respect to those who were gay. Now, two apparently "decent" men living together were regarded as homosexuals. The forty-year-old bachelor uncle was no longer seen as a mere eccentric.

The large number of gay people with AIDS ensured that the names of the majority of gays were revealed. Each person who became ill and died left a string of friends and acquaintances who were now linked together by their sexual orientation. Costa Rican homosexuals were forced out of the closet by the pandemic.

For a small country and an even smaller gay population, the epidemic was to have a devastating effect. From 1983 to July 1998, 923 homosexual and bisexual men developed the disease. If we factor in the 30 to 50 percent of unreported cases, another 276 to 461 individuals contracted the disease without the authorities being notified. Each year, between twenty-six and 127 homo-bisexual men developed the disease. During this period, 506 have died, approximately two homo-bisexual men each week.[18] The link between AIDS and the gay community, which accounted for more than 67 percent of all cases until 1996, revealed sexual orientation.

The trauma of losing nearly 1,000 people and the fact that thousands of others were infected with the virus were to have a great impact on Costa Rica's gay community and on the way in which it related to the heterosexual majority. Homosexuals realized that Latin-style concealment and pretense was no longer of any use. The epidemic seemed likely to spread unchecked given the government's unwillingness to launch a prevention campaign. In fact, the government's initial response was to increase the number of raids and create panic about AIDS.

Because of the spread of AIDS among the gay population, on April 5, 1987, the Health Ministry decided to raid the bar La Torre, the most popular gay discotheque at the time, with the aim of "preventing" the epidemic.

> Hundreds of gays were taken off to jail without protest. Some later said that they felt like Jews being taken to the slaughterhouse: the ironic smiles of the police, being treated like criminals, the Deputy Interior Minister Ramos directing and observing the events and enjoying the degrading spectacle.[19]

Unlike Stonewall in the United States, there was no riot that night, or the next night, or any night so far. But things changed. For the first time in the country's history, gays and lesbians joined together to form the first political organization, and they protested to the media about the raid. From this movement, several political organizations and anti-AIDS groups were to emerge, such as prevention programs and a series of gay institutions and businesses that are the equal of any in the major Latin American cities.

The objective of the Association for the Fight Against AIDS, founded in 1987, and ILPES, founded in 1993, was to prevent AIDS in the community, a task that the government was unwilling to undertake. Beginning that year, prevention and awareness courses were programmed for gays with the aim of encouraging safe sex.

Promoting safe sex implied something more than simply using a condom. In the session on safer sex (the workshops consist of twelve three-hour sessions), the facilitators encourage participants to consider forms of sexual contact that do not involve penetration. One of the exercises, for example, involves imagining what would happen if men did not have genitals but still wanted to have sexual relations. Another session explores the value of masturbation as complete sex.

Oral sex is encouraged as a safe alternative (despite the debate on the issue). So are homosexual pornographic films. However, one of the most important issues discussed is Christian guilt and the persecution of homosexuality. The workshops try to analyze why the Christian Church persecutes gays and how they are made invisible and harassed by an arbitrary sexual morality.

About 3,000 gay and bisexual men have attended ILPES workshops.[20] In a small community, this is a substantial figure, because the information, the questions, and the different options are shared with others, and the ideas are disseminated beyond the official number of participants.

The workshops not only served to encourage the organization of the gay community but also questioned the excessive importance attached to penetration in the Latin culture. As one of the facilitators told us, "It was time that we Latins stopped thinking that sex was just fucking."

In the 1989 survey, we found that penetration was the preferred sexual practice. Of 162 gay men who frequented bars and were selected at random, only 23 percent admitted to feeling very excited about fellating a man wearing a condom. If a condom was not used, the number increased to 48 percent. When asked about active anal penetration, 41 percent admitted to feeling very excited with a condom and 64 percent without a condom. In other words, nearly double preferred penetration to oral sex.[21]

THE BODY REVOLUTION

Despite the gays' growing political organization in the country, by 1998 the members of all these groups numbered barely 100 people. For a generation that grew up in the 1960s and 1970s, it was not easy to be openly gay in such a small country as Costa Rica. Since social repression remains overwhelming, the majority of gays who have taken the courses are still fearful of exposing themselves through political participation. However, AIDS continues to have an impact on them. On one hand, the workshops provided them the theory to question the prevailing model of penetration in the country. On the other, homosexual pornography would show them the practice.

According to Gary W. Dowsett, some studies in the United States suggest that organization and participation in the gay community are not important factors in explaining changes in safe sex.[22] However, participation was defined as interest or activism in gay organizations. In Australia, by contrast, participation was considered to include not only the political, but also the social and the sexual aspects. In other words, participation did not simply mean militancy, but also included people who socialized in bars and in public places known to be homosexual venues. When this information was included, it was discovered that the most important factor in explaining the reduction of unsafe sex was the degree of participation in the gay community.[23]

The reluctance of social scientists to include nonpolitical activities in the gay community under the heading of "organization" has led them to overlook the important changes brought about by social and sexual centers. Carrier, for example, believes that in Guadalajara little has changed in the lives of gays in recent years, since the number of homosexual bars and organizations has remained static.[24] In their study on homosexuality in the Dominican Republic, Antonio de Moya and Rafael Garcia also measure the impact of AIDS by the decrease in the number of gay bars and hotels.[25]

In Costa Rica, as in Australia, gay meeting centers experienced a kind of "sexual revolution of desire." Instead of decreasing in number, they actually increased, and instead of becoming more furtive they became more obvious. Bars and social centers have proliferated in recent years. Whereas in 1989 there were just four bars, three saunas, and no hotels exclusively for gays, by 1998 the figure had risen to twenty, including three new hotels.[26] However, Costa Rican homosexuals made enormous changes in their practices and sexual fantasies, which are not only evident in the number of public or private establishments. Unlike what was reported in Mexico by Carrier or in Santo Domingo by de Moya and Garcia, where AIDS traumatized and reduced the gay spaces, in Costa Rica the opposite occurred. One possible explanation for this difference is that the gay community here was able to mount an effective prevention campaign that would save it from imminent disaster and give it a sense of confidence in itself and in its ability to change things.

In the 1989 survey, during the first five years of the AIDS epidemic, gay people had already begun to make changes in their sexual practices. Men who went to bars had reduced or eliminated various practices with casual or occasional partners (those who were not steady partners) and had decreased the frequency of penetration by the following percentages:

Active anal penetration:	34 percent
Passive anal penetration:	37 percent

At the same time, masturbation had increased significantly in 60 percent of cases, and 40 percent had never had oral sex.[27]

The reports from the prevention workshops clearly show that there was a period of panic during the early years of the epidemic, when gays preferred to rent porn videos and masturbate at home rather than make contacts in bars or public places. However, after a gradual acceptance of the condom and with the knowledge gained from workshops and movies, they opted to make changes. According to Carlos, a workshop participant, "The first years were very difficult for me. I was terrified of AIDS and of getting infected. I preferred to have sex alone. However, as I began to feel comfortable with safe sex, I began to enjoy it again and to go out to bars and public places." Ernesto confirms that "pornography was my teacher. That's how I learned to enjoy things other than penetration. I remember that before it had never occurred to me to do other things. Semen disgusted me and I didn't like oral sex. However, I learned new things and I began to enjoy them. You get used to everything." In Pepe's case, change was easier: " I joined the gay scene when there was AIDS and it was more common to masturbate and have oral sex than before. I started off in a different school from those who had become gay before the epidemic."

After the initial "shock" of the gays, at a time when people were still unaware of the danger of contagion through oral sex, information that oral sex was not dangerous, even without the protection of a condom, was a factor that propelled a kind of sexual revolution. Both masturbation and oral sex would become the safest and most favored practices in occasional relations and, even more important, would be performed according to scripts learned from pornography in public places. During a period that is difficult to pinpoint exactly, but within the past ten years, homosexuality stopped imitating the Latin heterosexual model with its emphasis on penetration, discretion, shame, and double standards.[28] The longstanding pact with the Church and the State was coming to an end: the practice of homosexuality would come out of the closet and become public in the very heart of the city. Moreover, things would not be done in accordance with the traditional Latin model, which considers only penetration as true sex. From now on, oral sex and masturbation would be the preferred practices. This would bring enormous benefits: from 1995, the number of new AIDS cases among gay and bisexual men was to decline sharply.[29]

Obviously, the changes were not general: there is always a vanguard group who leads the way. Not all gays learned from porn movies, nor did everyone use public places, as we shall see farther on. However, a larger number of gays began to "take over" these places and turn them into a kind of school for sexuality. Others used them to work on aspects of their personalities implanted during childhood. For whatever reasons, neither the places nor the gays would ever be the same.

Homosexual pornographic films, which can be viewed comfortably at home, are mainly imported from the United States. Unlike traditional Latin American culture, they have other values:

1. Language is minimal and the dialogues are simply a pretext for sex. Even when there is dialogue, it is in English and most Costa Ricans do not understand it.
2. Oral sex acquires great importance. The actors show how it is done and appear to enjoy doing it for long periods. In some videos, the whole sexual encounter is based on this practice.
3. Group sex, masturbation, voyeurism, and a certain sadism are promoted. Actors enjoy watching others have sex, through drapes, peepholes, or telescopes.
4. It is important to show men ejaculating. Porno movies convince viewers that the movie is real by the careful filming of ejaculation. However, not everyone ejaculates at the same time, showing that there is no reason for synchronization.
5. The action is filmed in particular locations; nontraditional spaces, such as public places, are chosen.

6. There is a degree of expectation and even danger in not knowing the sexual orientation of the actors. Part of the eroticism is the seduction of men who are apparently not identifiable as gay.
7. Size confers power. The male sexual organ is large. If it were not of generous proportions, the actor would not find work. The man with the largest penis is usually the one who penetrates or receives oral sex.
8. Masculinity is privileged. The actors are macho. North American porno movies exclude effeminate men.
9. Physical beauty brings benefits. Although porn movie actors are generally attractive, the best-looking ones receive more attention from the cameras and from other actors.

These are the rules that are followed in public places, as we shall see in the following chapters. Ironically, what began as a change in the gay sexual culture and did away with the implicit understanding that homosexual practice should be hidden from public view has brought changes to nonhomosexual communities.

Chapter 1

Methodology of the Study

FIRST STUDY (1989)

In 1989, we conducted a study of gay men to determine the risk factors for HIV infection.[1] This study was divided into two main areas. One part covered the quantitative aspects; in other words, a survey by quota sample was applied to different groups of men who have sex with men, through the use of a structured questionnaire. The other part consisted of an ethnographic study, directed at groups that were difficult to reach and that frequented public sex places such as saunas, parks, movie theaters, and public toilets. This study is used to make comparisons between the situation in 1989 and that in 1998. Observations were carried out in public places and in-depth interviews were conducted with clients.

For this work, we recruited a gay man who had researched these activities and who served as a participatory observer, in-depth interviewer, and analyst of the situation in four specific types of places: parks and alleyways, public toilets, movie theaters, and saunas. Over a period of three months, the ethnographer participated in activities in these areas and, without revealing his identity as a researcher, collected information. Every day he recorded the activities in each place and the nonstructured interviews carried out with clients, which would then be transcribed. Given that the schedule of activities in each place was different, the ethnographer was able to go to the movie theaters and saunas in the afternoons, and concentrate on the parks, alleyways, and derelict buildings at night.

We considered it necessary to keep his work secret for several reasons. In the first place, if had he disclosed his role as an observer he would have aroused suspicion, apprehension, and mistrust, which in turn would have distorted the information gathered. In the second place, because some of these places are extremely dangerous, anyone regarded as extraneous to the activities taking place could be the target of attacks. This happened in any case, since the ethnographer was assaulted on two occasions. In the case of the in-depth interviews, the ethnographer did explain the purpose of the study to the interviewees. We did not include their names or any data that might identify them.

Most of the interviews were conducted with gay men who had attended AIDS-prevention workshops at the Association for the Fight Against AIDS (a nongovernmental organization that later became ILPES), who volunteered to be interviewed and who admitted to having had sex in public places. However, it was later possible to carry out short interviews in the parks and saunas with men who had not attended the workshops. These short interviews were included in the analysis carried out by the ethnographer. However, the in-depth interviews were analyzed independently from the ethnographer's reports and were divided as follows:

- *Saunas:* a total of twenty-two in-depth interviews were carried out in situ over a three-month period. In addition, the ethnographer made ten three-hour visits to each of the saunas studied.
- *Parks:* twenty short interviews, lasting between half an hour and an hour, were conducted with clients, all of them gay men recruited from the AIDS-prevention workshops provided by the Association for the Fight Against AIDS. The ethnographer also carried out fifty hours of observation over a three-month period.
- *Public toilets, alleyways, and empty buildings:* ten gay clients were interviewed in these places who also attended AIDS-prevention workshops. No interviews were carried out in the PSPs (public sex places), but rather in clients' homes. The ethnographer spent a total of forty hours at the selected points over a three-month period.
- *Movie theaters:* By appointment, ten gay men who frequented movie theaters for sex were interviewed in cafes or at home. These men volunteered during AIDS-prevention workshops to be interviewed. The interviews lasted approximately two hours each. In addition, the ethnographer spent twenty hours at a selected movie theater over a three-month period.

SECOND STUDY (1998)

The 1998 study was called "Public Sex Places." The investigation was undertaken by the Research Department of the Latin American Institute for Prevention and Health Education, ILPES, in the metropolitan area of San José.

The study was directed by chief researcher Dr. Jacobo Schifter, Regional Director of ILPES, assisted by a general coordinator, Rodrigo Vargas, who, in addition to supervising the different phases of the study, was also responsible for drafting the various guides and questionnaires used in the study, together with other team members and under the supervision of Dr. Schifter.

Objective

The general objective of the study was to update our information on the activities taking place in public sex places, eight years after the first survey.

Public sex places are defined as all areas accessible to the public, such as parks, spas, public lavatories, saunas, study centers, movie theaters, and massage parlors, both indoor and outdoor establishments, frequented by men who have sex with other men and who use these places to make contacts or have sexual relations.

Work Schedule

The first phase of the process included preparation of the research plan, the development of research tools and the sample design, the selection of the actual sample, and the hiring and training of interviewers and of the staff collaborating in the application of the in-depth interview guides, guides for ethnographic observation, and the questionnaires. This phase lasted approximately two months.

The second phase, consisting of fieldwork, lasted two months. At the same time, a database was developed to enter the information from the questionnaires, and the interviews were transcribed. This process, in its entirety, lasted four months.

Finally, the third phase included the treatment and presentation of the data (tabulation and preparation of the transcriptions of the in-depth interviews) and the drafting of the final report to the research director for subsequent analysis.

Given the fact that men who have sex with other men are found in all social, cultural, and geographic spheres, it was necessary to extend the geographic boundaries of public sex places in the metropolitan area of San José to include a particular location outside the city, because of its importance.

In 1989, we had discovered the presence of three main protagonists in public sex places: gay men, sex workers, and police officers. By 1998 it was decided that the ethnographic study should also include in-depth interviews with these three groups, and therefore three general coordinators were appointed to conduct interviews with each group and observe their different roles.

THE QUANTITATIVE STUDY

In the 1998 study we wanted to test some of the hypotheses on the reasons for visiting public places for sex. To obtain a representative sample, we decided to select men who frequent homosexual social centers in the city of San José. Our idea was to carry out the survey with the objective of making subsequent comparisons. Once the data had been analyzed, our population of gay men would be divided into those who visited public places to have sexual relations and those who did not, and we would then try to examine the similarities and differences between them.

A questionnaire was designed with the objective of gathering the necessary information to determine the possible reasons why people frequent public places to have sexual relations. Most of the questionnaire was structured and precodified, and contained approximately ninety questions divided into the following sections: identification of the interview, social and demographic variables, sexual self-definition and people who are familiar with sexual self-definition, first sexual experience, sexual relations and couples, sexual communication, violence, visits to public sex places and motivations, condom use and consumption of alcohol and drugs in public sex places, family background, emotional, physical, and sexual abuse, self-perception, and questions for the interviewer. The duration of the interviews are shown in Table 1.1.

TABLE 1.1. Data Relating to Duration of the Interviews

	(N) (301) Total 100
Duration of interview	**Percentage**
Less than 20 minutes	27.6
20-24	29.6
25-29	16.9
30-34	11.6
35 and over	14.3
Statistics related to duration of interview	**Values**
Average	23.6
Mode	20.0
Median	22.0
Minimum	10.0
Maximum	85.0

The survey was carried out by a team of five interviewers who had received prior training. The process lasted approximately four weeks and no major problems were encountered during the survey. The quantitative study was carried out with a population of men who have sex with other men and who frequented social areas located in the metropolitan area of San José at the time of the survey.

In theory, this means that the sample consists of homosexual men who participate in Costa Rica's gay community and leaves out those who frequent PSPs but do not participate in gay social centers. However, as we shall see later, the fact of participating in social centers or not doing so does not have the same significance in a Latin country as it does in the United States.

These social centers or meeting points were defined as places or commercial establishments such as bars, restaurants, or discotheques that are frequented mainly by men who have sex with other men. Bearing in mind the obvious limitations of time and resources, we decided to concentrate the survey in these places, since access was relatively easy. Once we had compiled a list of all these establishments, of the days and hours when they were open and of the number of clients who came daily or nightly, we proceeded to prepare the sample design and finally the sample itself.

To select the sample, there was no existing sample design that would permit us to establish a process of selection. Nevertheless, it was feasible to build one.

In doing so, the following steps were taken:

1. A list of bars, saloons, discotheques, and restaurants frequented by the target population was prepared.
2. A preliminary interview with the owner or manager of each establishment was arranged to introduce the study and secure their collaboration.
3. The list of social meeting places had to include the days on which the establishment was open, the hours when it was open, and an approximate number of clients who visited daily or nightly. In some cases, the number of clients was rather difficult to calculate, especially in larger establishments such as restaurants and discotheques. For this reason, it was indispensable to secure the collaboration of the owner or manager to obtain the most precise data possible.

The sample design included a total of seven establishments with the required characteristics.

To find out whether the sample was viable, an estimate was made of the number of visitors to the establishments on the days they were open. The results indicated that it was possible to obtain the sample size required. We stress that these estimates were made for the sole purpose of assessing the possibility of securing the required sample size. The estimates cannot represent an exact number of clients since the people who frequent these places are not always the same, nor do they arrive with the same frequency. In addition, the opening hours of these places differ and the number of visitors can fluctuate due to the opening or closure of these centers.

Once we had constructed the sample design, the next step was to determine how many interviews would be carried out at each establishment. Given that we obtained a list of establishments with an approximate number of visitors per day, the sample was proportionally assigned to this variable.

The random nature of the sample was determined by the choice of hours at random and because it was considered that the flow of people who visit a specific establishment also occurs randomly. In fact the selection of certain specific hours at random was done for reasons of order and to avoid a situation where the interviewer would have a heavy work load that he could not handle.

Finally, 301 interviews were carried out at the different social centers. In this case, the sampling procedure was applied with probability proportional to the size of the establishment (number of people visiting a given place—PPS). The size of the sample was determined, taking account of the time necessary to obtain results and availability of funds.

In general, the degree of cooperation encountered during the interviews was acceptable, since 95.3 percent of the interviewers described it as good or very good. Moreover, 87 percent of the interviewers described the results in the same way.

THE QUALITATIVE STUDY

This book is also based on two other, additional sources: the ethnographic observation and the in-depth interviews.

In the first case, an ethnographic observation guide was applied to study the culture of the people who frequent public sex places, which entailed living with them day by day. Specifically, we studied behavioral patterns, the "rules of the game," high-risk sexual practices, and the types of contacts that occur in the places.

To this end, observations were conducted in ten parks, five saunas, three movie theaters, a university, four public toilets, one video club, one spa, one alleyway, and one fast-food restaurant. This process continued for one month in each place.

During the second phase, sixty in-depth interviews were carried out with public sex clients over a period of approximately three months. For the purposes of this study, the clients included gay men, sex workers, and even police officers, who also participate in public sex, as we shall see later. Subsequently, we requested forty written accounts from gay men with a history of sexual and physical abuse.

Ethnographic Observation

We conducted in-depth interviews or received written accounts as follows:

1. Gay clients of PSPs (twenty interviews)
2. Gay men at abuse workshops (forty written accounts)
3. Sex workers (twenty interviews)
4. Police officers (twenty interviews)

It is important to note that in the places studied, identities are fluid and therefore differentiation is not always easy. A policeman may turn into a *cachero* or a sex worker, a "locust" may move from crime to prostitution (these terms are defined later), a prostitute may become a criminal, and a gay can end up as a prostitute.

Gay Men Who Are Clients in PSPs

Gay men are an important sector of the clients in PSPs. Some participate in the gay community (bars, discotheques, organizations) and others do not.

We conducted twenty in-depth interviews, lasting two hours, with gay men who attended AIDS-prevention workshops organized by ILPES and who frequent public sex places. Abelardo Araya, coordinator of the organization's gay program, was responsible for securing the voluntary participation of workshop participants who visit PSPs and for carrying out the interviews. These included a series of questions about the interviewees' life history, family background, relationships with parents, family violence, homosexuality and homophobia, reasons for frequenting public sex places, sexual practices, risk of HIV infection, drug use, and other related issues.

The fact that participants in the AIDS-prevention workshops should be our main source of information implies that these homosexuals share a certain degree of recognition of their sexual identity. However, this recognition is not of the same type that exists in the United States. For a Latin "gay," being out of the closet is more a question of inwardly accepting his own sexuality, rather than expressing it to the rest of the world. In other words, it is an end to the mental repression of his own homosexuality.[2] Coming "out of the closet" does not imply activism or open participation. Thus, many of the gays who are out of the closet in Costa Rica are actually hidden, and the difference between those who believe they are out and those who do not is only a matter of degree.

Nevertheless, for the purposes of this study and analysis of the results, it is important to point out that the gay sector, which is in theory more open and more involved in Costa Rica's gay community, is most strongly represented. This leaves out a group who frequent public places but who are not clients of gay bars and who do not participate in homosexual organizations.

Gay Men with a History of Sexual and Physical Abuse

One group with whom we worked in a different way were gay men with a history of sexual and physical abuse. When we analyzed the survey and found that the violence and sexual abuse factor was so significant, we decided to conduct an additional exploration of the links between visiting public sex places and a previous history of physical and sexual violence.

Since ILPES had programmed a series of workshops between September and November 1998 for men who had suffered physical or sexual abuse, we decided to search for answers among the participants. Approximately forty men participated in these workshops, which were held independently of this study. Participation was completely voluntary. ILPES had invited clinical psychologists to refer some of their patients who were interested in working on their abuse experiences with a group of gay men, under the supervision of psychologists specializing in this area. An announcement was also posted to enable those who had attended ILPES' AIDS-prevention workshops to participate.

To understand the relationship between violence and participation in public sex places, we obtained permission to recruit four workshop participants who wished to contribute to our study. Their role was to introduce to each of the four groups, three tasks or assignments relating to sexual and physical abuse and participation in public sex places. We obtained anonymous copies of the accounts written by the participants on: the sexual abuse they had suffered, their most erotic encounters in public places, and their own analyses of the similarities and differences they saw in both cases.

Of the forty participants, twenty-three frequented public sex places. We selected only the accounts of clients of these places and have included five of them in this study. Although they contain experiences and analyses that are common to all twenty-three cases, we believe that the interpretation of the relationship between abuse and public sex places should be studied with a much broader and more representative population. These analyses should therefore be considered speculative and as possible subjects for further study.

Cacheros, Chapulines, and Criminals

The interviews with men involved in prostitution were conducted at El Salon, a project for sex workers and criminals in the center of San José, with the support of project director Antonio Bustamante, who provided us with a list of young men who are criminals and were willing to be interviewed. The interviews were conducted by ILPES journalist Dino Starcevic.

This ILPES project works with various groups of men who are involved in prostitution and crime, mainly robbery: *cacheros*, common criminals, and *chapulines* or "locusts." The differences and similarities between these groups make it difficult to categorize them.

In the book *Lila's House*, we define *cachero* as a man who, in Latin sexual culture, is perceived as the penetrator in anal sex with another man, and who is therefore not regarded as a homosexual.[3] In his work on homosexuality in Mexico, Carrier tells us that in Mexico this figure is known as the *mayate.*[4] In the Dominican Republic, according to de Moya and Garcia, *cacheros* are known as *bugarrones.*[5] *Cacherismo* has a long history in Costa Rica and is practiced by heterosexual men who, for different reasons, do not have access to women (prison inmates, banana and coffee plantation workers, sailors, truck drivers, and others). However, the category *cachero* is more fluid than many people realize and there are *cacheros* who are involved in prostitution in marginal areas. *Cacheros* also engage in more varied sexual practices than they admit to.[6]

Cacheros who engage in prostitution are not homosexuals in the "modern" sense of the word. Studies on male prostitution in the United States suggest that most of them are not homosexuals either.

According to Coombs, the majority of young male prostitutes in the United States are typically masculine and heterosexual. The statistics for his sample of 124 individuals are: 6 percent homosexual, 22 percent bisexual, and 72 percent heterosexual.[7] Similar results were obtained in Denmark, where Jersild, in a study of 300 male prostitutes in Copenhagen, identified only six as homosexuals.[8] In his study on male prostitution, Ginsburg expresses the view that the homosexual act does not make an individual gay and notes that most of the sex workers he interviewed were not homosexuals, though he recognizes that some of them might become so through practice.[9]

Some believe that the practice of *cacherismo* is a convenient category invented by men in homophobic societies to "escape" the stigma of homosexuality. Others, such as Rudi C. Bleys, believe that not considering *cacheros* as homosexuals is part of the tradition of European ethnography which, since the nineteenth century, has considered those who are effeminate to be homosexuals, but not so those who are masculine.[10] However, our own studies show that this category does not serve to protect *cacheros* from discrimination. Among the middle classes, for example, *cacheros* are regarded as homosexuals both by heterosexuals and by homosexuals themselves. However, among the lower social classes, the heterosexual identity of the *cachero* is accepted among people of all sexual orientations. This tolerance is a reflection of a sexual culture that considers practice to be more important than the sexual object in determining sexual identity. The sexual culture of certain sectors of Latino culture focuses more on the body to define the sexuality of a person: men are men so long as they are "active" sexually, whether with women, men, children, or animals.[11]

The group of nongay men who frequent public sex places consists mainly of *cacheros* involved in prostitution. In other words, these are men who have sex with other men for money. Unlike other types of *cacheros*, such as prison inmates or sailors, they are not interested in sexual satisfaction. As was shown in *Lila's House*, *cacheros* who are prostitutes are not sexually attracted to their clients, have not had a history of sex with men prior to working in the sex trade, and do not consider themselves to be homosexuals. Most of them have sex with women and have fathered children.[12]

Not all prostitutes are *cacheros*, nor are all *cacheros* prostitutes. As we shall see, public sex places are also frequented by homosexual prostitutes, in other words, sex workers who *are* attracted to other men, who define themselves as gay, and who make money from sex. However, homosexual prostitutes and *cacheros* do not share the same sexual identity and are concerned that they should not be perceived as doing so. For this reason, they even position themselves in different areas or sections of the public sex places. Other *cacheros*, such as former prison inmates or police officers, also frequent public sex places to satisfy themselves sexually and do not engage in prostitution.

In the list provided to us by the director of El Salon, prostitutes included *chapulines* or "locusts" as well as *cacheros*. The locusts are juvenile delinquents who steal and work in gangs. These gangs emerged fairly recently and their modus operandi is to mug and rob people in Costa Rican cities. The term locusts was coined only ten years ago. Some locusts are as young as eight or nine years old, while others are over thirty. However, the majority are teenagers. The members of these young criminal gangs caught our interest because now they are also working as prostitutes in public sex places. These young criminals who engage in prostitution also appear in studies conducted in the United States. In his study on male prostitution, Gandy included what he termed "hoodlum hustlers or heterosexual delinquents"[13] while Raven mentions the "smart, small time crook who sees the homosexual as an easy mark."[14] Despite their differences, these groups are similar to Costa Rica's *chapulines*, in that they are more criminals than prostitutes. In the Dominican Republic, de Moya and Garcia mention groups of adolescents involved in prostitution and theft, known as *palomos*.[15] However, the *palomos* are more involved in prostitution than in mugging people in the cities.

Approximately 150 *cacheros*, locusts, and delinquents attend the El Salon project each week. Out of the twenty who were interviewed, thirteen described themselves as locusts, and the rest as delinquents. None of them described themselves as homosexual, bisexual, or "gay," though eighteen admitted to having had sexual relations with men. Their initiation into homosexual sex took place within the terms of prostitution, and none admitted to feeling desire or having fantasies about other men. When they were asked directly about how they viewed their sexual relations with other men, the general reply was as *cacheros* (not all of them used this word, but used similar terms such as "male-men," "macho," or "male"), in other words, acts that take place between "men" (heterosexuals) and homosexuals. In their accounts, the interviewees did not admit to being penetrated by clients, but they did recognize that "other locusts" had done it for money.

The program coordinators are both heterosexuals and homosexuals, although ILPES is known for its work with homosexuals. In view of this reputation, it is possible that those who attend El Salon are the *cacheros* and locusts who are most involved in prostitution. This could be a subject for future study.

Public sex places are also frequented by common criminals who are not locusts. Some of them are *cacheros* and others are simply there to rob people. It is hard to tell them apart. Both the common criminals and the *cacheros* try to pick men up with the aim of robbing them or charging them for sex. However, many criminals end up having sex with their potential victims and many *cacheros* end up robbing their clients. Although some of the interviewees described themselves as common delinquents—muggers and thieves who work alone—they were not the focus of our study. The similarities and differences between delinquents and locusts should be analyzed in a future study.

Members of El Salon who offered themselves as volunteers were given a two-hour in-depth interview. The following subjects were discussed: personal and family background of the interviewee, first sexual experiences and sexual desire, public sex places, sexual self-definition of the interviewee, sexual orientation and homosexuality, prostitution and sexual culture in public sex places, money and prostitution, HIV/AIDS, other sexually transmitted diseases and prevention, violence, relations with the police, and consumption of tobacco, alcohol, and drugs.

Our interest centered on the thirteen interviewees who described themselves as locusts, since this is a criminal group which only recently began to practice *cacherismo* and because it is linked to several recent crimes against gay men. The fact that some of these crimes were perpetrated by several youths (common delinquents do not usually operate in gangs) suggests involvement by locusts. The fact that some of the locusts interviewed admit to having wounded or having been on the verge of killing some clients (though none admitted to actually perpetrating a crime) is another sign of their involvement. However, not all crimes against gays have been committed by locusts, nor are they all killers. Several of the common delinquents or "prostitute *cacheros*" interviewed admitted to having mugged or attacked gay men in public places. Some killings were committed by criminals who acted alone.

At the same time, the activities of locusts and prostitute *cacheros* may vary. Some of those in the first group are now more involved in prostitution than robbery. Some from the second group, when they age or lose their appeal, engage more in robbery than in prostitution. Others change their activities for short periods, according to circumstances. When there are more tourists in town, for example, they engage in prostitution with foreigners, and when there are fewer tourists they rob local people.

Finally, once the interviews had been analyzed, an extra session was held with ten locusts who admitted to having attacked their clients. We asked this group to help us interpret or "read the story" of three crimes against gays. The extra session lasted approximately one hour with each interviewee.

Police Officers

Twenty in-depth interviews were conducted with police officers based at the police stations close to the public sex places in the study, and with officers on the university campus, those in patrol cars, and members of the mounted police units who patrol the parks. Police commanders were asked to supply a list of police officers and were asked for permission to interview officers who patrol the public sex places. The person in charge of making these contacts and conducting the interviews was Luis Villalta, coordinator of an ILPES program for former prison inmates, in close collaboration with the Ministry of Justice. Among the issues discussed were personal and family background, sexual practices and behavior, homosexuality, public sex places, HIV/AIDS, other sexually transmitted diseases and prevention, violence and human rights, and consumption of cigarettes, alcohol, and drugs.

The interviews were conducted in three police stations in San José, and lasted an average of three to five hours. These exchanges took place in fairly adverse conditions, because other police officers were constantly entering the room where they were held.

The police officers work at three police stations (whose names are not given for the protection of the interviewees), but cannot be considered representative of the San José police or even of the other officers at their stations. However, the fourteen officers who are based at these three stations were selected precisely because their superiors identified them as being in charge of security at the parks, movie theaters, and public toilets in the study. The other interviewees were assigned to the university campus (two), patrol cars (two), or the mounted police that patrolled the areas studied (two).

Several subjects were discussed with the police officers: social and demographic variables, family history and violence, ethics, perceptions of homosexuality, homophobia, work relations, and intervention in public sex places.

No payments were made for the interviews with the police officers or the gays. The participants of the El Salon project each received a $10 fee for the interview.

Chapter 2

The Geography of Desire: 1989

When we began our ethnographic study, we found a small and unspecialized world. Nine years ago, public sex places could be counted on the fingers of your hands, and people invested a fair amount of time in making contacts. The number of participants was relatively small for a country with a metropolitan area of more than one million inhabitants. Moreover, sexual encounters were more a question of individuals than groups and were carried out with some discretion. Below is a summary of the reports provided by ethnographers and eyewitnesses.

THE PARKS AND SURROUNDING AREAS

The Parque Monumental is located just east of downtown San José. It was built at the end of the nineteenth century in the place formerly known as the Plaza de la Liberal (Freedom Square). It consists of two acres of land planted with trees. Some are huge fig trees, more than fifty years old, with enormous roots that struggle to invade new territory. Unlike European parks, there is no pattern or order in the size, type, or shape of the trees. A pine tree, a fig tree, a mango tree, and a eucalyptus stand side by side. "The trees here are planted by birds who shit the seeds," says Ernesto, a high school student. The Municipality of San José is responsible for the park's upkeep, but seems content to send in the gardeners once or twice a year. "When they come here," adds Ernesto, "they do such a quick cleanup that you don't know if the place was hit by lightning or if they pruned the trees." It's not clear whether the gardeners use fertilizer. "The only fertilizer these trees get is the piss from old queens and kids who come here to fuck," says our interviewee. The stench of urine among the tree roots confirms his assertions. "The queens do wonders for these trees. Since they drink so much liquor and do so much crack, they feed the soil. These trees are well fertilized with coke. Don't tell me that crack doesn't make plants grow!" he remarks.

In the center of the park stands a monument to Costa Rica's heroes. Bronze statues of well-built men hold the national flag aloft in military triumph. "This is an important monument because it represents the battle in which Costa Ricans prevented the country's annexation to the United States," we are told by a man who frequents this park. "Was the United States really going to invade Costa Rica?" we ask with curiosity. "Well, not the government directly, but a few gringo bandits led from Nicaragua," adds a sex worker.[1] "The gringos have always wanted to invade us and fuck us Ticos," he adds. "Well, in the end they didn't succeed," we say to continue the conversation. "Yeah, but now they come here and fuck queens behind this monument," he says with indignation. "Anyway," he adds, "what the hell did we gain with independence? Us poor people didn't gain anything. They'd pay us more in Miami to give our asses to foreigners than what we get here."

Cement benches *(poyos)* are distributed throughout the park. The park is designed in the landscaped architectural style characteristic of the turn of the century. "These benches are so hard—they leave you with a flat ass," complains a student, who uses them during the day to study. "And they're so old and damp and full of mold. Here it rains six months of the year and the benches get wet every day and nobody cleans them. Well, you need to clean them before you sit down. Can't you see how careless people are? They spill their soda all over the seats." The innocent student does not realize that she has sat on a semen stain left from the night before.

Except for the steps leading up to the monument, the benches are the only places to sit. There are about eighty of them around the park. Some are closer to sidewalks that surround the park, while others are hidden among the leafy trees. "This is my favorite bench," says a gay who comes to this park at night. "It has a beautiful view and is very well positioned. It's also very discreet because it's covered by a branch that fell about a year ago. I need to get here early because there's a bunch of queens who try to grab it from me. In this country, nobody respects other people's property. When I go I leave a few thumbtacks so that the next queen who sits here will get stuck in the ass."

Although Parque Monumental has artificial lighting, much of it is often in darkness because of electrical problems that last several days. According our interviewee Mario, a seventeen-year-old student:

> The behavior of the groups who come to the park has a lot to do with the lighting. What happens here is determined by whether or not the area is lit, or whether it's daytime or nighttime. The fact that there is no lighting encourages some people to enter the park to make their contacts and others to fuck with other people. It's very interesting to see how when it's dark, people are a bit freer, in the sense that they can openly participate in sex, even with penetration. Sometimes the darkness provides cover for folks to have orgies with three to five people.

When the park is well lit, people are more restrained and, though they will pick up partners at a bench or as they walk, it is done with more caution. People approach each other, greet each other, and say a few introductory words to get to know each other a little. "Gays are the enemies of lighting," adds Mario. "There's a whole tradition of smashing street lights here. There's a famous queen who's known as the baseballer because she goes around breaking them. Some couples will even pay her to break a lamp."

But the park is not the only pickup point. There are nearby alleyways which, because they are in permanent darkness, become very crowded. "The parks have their own roots, like the trees," says Eduardo, another gay client. "In other words, they spread out into the surrounding alleyways, empty houses, or vacant lots."

This is the case of an alleyway that is located near a public institution. It is used by couples who meet in the park and who are looking for a little more privacy. It is a dark place that runs diagonally across the block, behind a large public building. There is an exit at both ends of the alleyway, and the railroad line passes along one side. "A lot of queens like to fuck in this alleyway. They're known as the locomotives because they like to play "little trains" right on the railroad lines. One day they're all going to get flattened together," says Carlos, a twenty-eight-year-old gay who is a regular here.

The other side of the alleyway is flanked by the garden walls of a few houses. It is a foul-smelling place because of the indigents who defecate by the walls and the large heaps of garbage dumped by local residents. During certain times of the year, the grass grows tall and needs to be cut regularly.

Gay activity begins at nightfall. There is already a fair amount of action between 6 and 6:30 in the evening. Unlike the park, the clientele here is predominantly gay and the area is less exposed to passersby.

About two blocks away from the park is a bus stop with a very popular public toilet. Though the urinal measures only six feet square and is unlit, it is a busy venue for public sex during the day, and especially at night.

In the daytime, a young man charges people two colones (in 1989) to use the urinal. This measure was introduced by the authorities as a way of controlling the intense sexual activity. But after 6 p.m. the attendant leaves and the place becomes a pickup point and a place for sexual encounters.

This particular toilet has become a well-known place for gay sex. On several occasions the ethnographer heard a heterosexual man coming in to use the toilet, and because the urinal was full of gays (eight people can squeeze in tightly), he was told: "Take a piss outside, because it's full of queers in there," or "Don't go in there because you'll get raped by the sodomites inside." He replied, "But I need to pee," to make the straight men reveal what was going on inside. "Well, you'd better pee into a Coke bottle," they answered, "because in that toilet they'll take out your milk and even your blood." When the man entered the toilet anyway, he heard them say "that sonofabitch is a sodomite too." This is how the ethnographer describes the toilet:

> The urinal stinks because nobody uses disinfectant here. Four men are inside pretending to urinate, but they are looking at other men's penises. Because I don't pee and stand watching the men, one says, "Well? What's the matter with you? This is

> a toilet and you don't come here to gawk." I answer firmly, "If this is a toilet, then what are you doing, 'cause I don't see anyone peeing." "Well, can't you see we've got our dicks out?" he says rudely. "Yeah, but I don't understand what you've got it out for if you just spend your time watching the guy next to you. Are you going to pee with his dick?" I ask them ironically. The other three begin to laugh and one turns around and touches my penis and says to the other, "Can't you see he's scared, and what he wants is for his daddy to help him piss." I decide to end the ethnographic observation and rush outside before he keeps his promise. However, the heterosexuals are still outside, pretending they're waiting to go in. "Did you have a good pee?" they yell mockingly.

Although the toilet closes after 11 or 11:30 at night, the ethnographer saw men masturbating each other and having oral sex outside the toilet, by the metal doors. "People don't come here to pee," says Eduardo. "This is a magical place where people know that you come to have sex, whether the doors are open or shut."

Three blocks away is a derelict house that was damaged by a fire. Alcoholics and people who live on the streets kicked down the door a couple of years ago. Apparently, the heirs to this property are involved in a lawsuit to determine who it belongs to. While the ponderous Costa Rican courts decide who the legitimate owner is, the park's clients have made it their second home. Because the house has no roof, it can only be used when it is not raining. However, the dividing walls of what used to be the three bedrooms, the lounge, the kitchen, and the entrance hall are still standing.

When you enter this house, only shadows are visible. Nevertheless, people have figured out a way to see who comes in: they strike a match or use a lighter, providing illumination for just a few brief seconds. Another method is to inhale on a cigarette. In this way, you can see the person who is next to you for just a few seconds and at the same time allow yourself to be seen. Juan, a young gay man of twenty-two, tells us that somebody once arrived with a flashlight. "People were really upset because it was like the police. This queen was shoving her flashlight in everyone's face. There was no privacy. The clients themselves broke her flashlight that night." The rule here is total darkness, interrupted only by the flicker of matches or the glow of cigarettes.

The house smells damp and pieces of burned wood lie scattered on the floor. When the ethnographer gets used to the darkness and the glow of cigarettes, he counts about half a dozen people. Half the clients are crammed into the entrance hall. He approaches and finds he is mistaken. Six of the men with cigarettes have partners who are giving them oral sex. Nobody seems bothered by his presence. One man inhales his cigarette and stares at him, while his partner kneels with his back to the ethnographer. The man inhales again and continues to stare at him. Although he is having sex with someone else, his interest is aroused by the ethnographer. He is a handsome and masculine man with beautiful eyes, and the ethnographer cannot avoid being attracted to him. "What is he thinking now that I'm looking at him?" he wonders. There is no ethnographical study that does not change the culture it observes.

MOVIE THEATERS

Other places frequented by gays in search of sexual contacts are movie theaters. One of these is located in the so-called red-light district, the most dangerous area of the capital. The movie theater is surrounded by brothels of women and transvestites. The building is old, dilapidated, and notoriously filthy inside. A sixty-year-old heavily made-up woman, who acts like a government bureaucrat, sells us tickets. We ask, "What time does the movie start?" "Don't worry, there are movies here all the time," she replies in an offhand manner. As she gives us our change, we ask ourselves whether this woman knows what goes on inside. The question is not easy to answer. Germans still argue about whether ordinary people knew what went on inside the concentration camps. Many victims of Treblinka who arrived at the camp from all over Europe would put on makeup and comb their hair before getting off the train. Although they had evidence that death awaited them, they fooled themselves until the very end. The human mind is a box of surprises and as the saying goes, "There is none so blind as he who will not see."

The movies are of poor quality, usually Mexican pictures or old box-office hits that are now very damaged. The tickets cost 440 colones. There are three shows, at 3, 7 and 9 p.m. Today they are showing an old Cantinflas movie (a popular Mexican comedian). The clients do not seem amused by the comic's antics. "The only thing we like about Cantinflas is that he walks around with his pants down," says a transvestite. "People only care about whether the movie is shot at night or in the daytime. If it's shot at night, there's less light and you can throw yourself at any man you want. When there's more light, you just look at people." In any case, Costa Rican humor is very different from Mexican humor and is even more remote for gays. "Costa Ricans don't have such a complex about being underdeveloped. Our problem is, we're not as developed as we think we are," remarks the transvestite.

The inside of the building is totally neglected. It smells of semen and urine. The seats are torn and some are broken. "Nobody is going to complain because they can't sit down," says Victor, a regular visitor to this place. "The truth is, the clients themselves break them with their orgies. This one was broken by Rhino, a fat queen who sat down on top of some punk. How can a poor piece of wood cope with a 220-pound whale who's leaping up and down like a squirrel in a tree?"

The people who come here have established different areas for sexual activity. As we shall see, the movie theater is divided into areas where different sexual practices take place and where different groups of homosexuals congregate, each one varying according to age, sexual desires, and social class. The clients have divided up the different sections in accordance with the divisions of the National Theater: circle, stalls, and balcony. However, the differences have nothing to do with proximity to or distance from the screen. "The balcony is the area that's darkest and farthest from the screen," says Victor.

The period before the movie begins is used by clients to look around for possible sexual contacts. When the lights go out, a general movement begins to the different areas of the theater. Victor, the ethnographer, says:

> Like I told you before, I think the Beirut is too cramped for so many people, but it's a gay place. Coming in here is none too

> pleasant because of its location—San José's red-light district. It's dirty from the beginning.

As you enter the building, the toilets are straight ahead and on the left is a staircase leading to the upper floor. The entrance to the theater is on the right. "You can hitch up in any of these places," says Victor. The whole area at the back of the theater is also an action point. According to Victor, it is "the area for the old guys who pay, who offer money to suck your dick or invite you out to eat if you'll go with them. I don't know how much they pay. They say it straight to your face: 'Hey, will you sleep with me today? I'll pay you something.'" We notice one or two older men leaving the building with a younger man. "Where do they go?" we ask our informer. "To seedy hotels nearby." "And how much do they pay these young kids?" we ask. "Well, not much, because the old guys don't have money. Some young guys will go with them because they don't have teeth and so they prefer them for oral sex. Here, having false teeth isn't considered a bad thing. On the contrary, some prostitutes refuse clients who have teeth."

Near the entrance to the theater, on the ground floor, are some filthy, fifty-year-old curtains, and behind them sit a group of men. Victor explains who they are. "They're the cock-sucking queens. They can see who goes into the bathroom, because you just pull the curtain a little and you can see who goes in. So these people sit there and as soon as someone goes to the bathroom, they get up and go see if they can suck him."

In this lower area, very close to the screen, is a door which is usually left half-open. The door leads directly to the bathroom. "This is where a lot of people sit to watch or to masturbate. . . . That area downstairs is dismal, completely dirty. You sit down and you can feel the lice biting. Everything makes you itch, like a kind of skin rash," says Alberto, Victor's friend. "People have sex there," continues Alberto, "but it's not so obvious. It's all hidden because the guy with the flashlight is there, so there's just a movement of hands, mutual masturbation and oral sex."

Upstairs, the theater is divided into three areas. The left-hand side is not too crowded, and few people sit in the central area. But on the right-hand side, which is hidden from view as you enter, "is Sodom and Gomorrah," exclaims Victor.

I sit in the upper circle and pretend to watch the movie. However, the real show is offscreen. A well-built man about thirty years old comes over and sits next to me. While Cantinflas acts the fool as a bullfighter on-screen, my new neighbor begins to touch me up and fixes his gaze on me. I'm afraid because I don't know what to do. I continue to look at the screen. While Cantinflas performs pirouettes, the guy takes out his penis and begins to touch it softly. Since I do not make any move, another man approaches him and places a coat on top of him. He puts his hand underneath and begins to masturbate him. Neither one says a word. Two employees with flashlights come by in search of a lost wallet. Although they pretend to fix their eyes on the floor, one says to the other, "This is the first time I see a coat dancing salsa."

SAUNAS

Saunas differ from the places mentioned previously because they are private establishments. The people who go there are exclusively homosexuals or bisexuals who know what kind of activities to expect. As far as the clientele is concerned, the men who frequent saunas are similar to those found in the bars: gay or bisexual men who prefer to be in places recognized as such. However, unlike the gay discotheques, the saunas have one purpose: sex. Moreover, as will be shown later, the type of man who goes to saunas is not necessarily the same as the one who go to bars.

For this part of the survey, we studied three gay saunas in San José. The first, known as Decoro, is located in downtown San José in an old, fairly dilapidated house. A small metal plaque on one side of the door is the only indication that this is a business. The entrance fee is 300 colones (in 1989) and the establishment opens at 2:00 in the afternoon and closes at 9:00 at night. It is run by the entire family of a gay married man: wife, mother, and son. When the mother is in charge, she behaves as if the place were really a spa. "Here's your towel and your soap, Sir, so you can have a good wash and stay healthy," says the mother, who wears a crucifix and has a statue of the Virgin in her small office. "Thank you very much," I reply. "Can you tell me what this sauna has?" I ask innocently. "Well, what would you expect it to have? A sauna, a bathroom, and a lounge," replies the woman irritably.

She herself cleans the cubicles and the bathrooms. "That old broad would have to be very dumb not to know what goes on inside. Sometimes she has to collect used condoms and dirty sheets. What does she think this is?" remarks a client who is not impressed by her apparent religious devotion.

On entering the premises, clients are handed a small blanket, a bath towel, and a padlock and key for their locker. They also pay their entrance fees.

As you begin to undress, you notice the difference from other public places. Here everyone knows what he is here for. There is no mystery, as in the parks and movie theaters. Nudity and desire are totally evident. Nevertheless, a certain Latin modesty persists. For example, two gay men wrap towels around themselves before taking off their underpants, thereby hiding their genitals. Others, however, undress completely before putting on a towel. "The guys who wrap towels around themselves before getting undressed usually have small dicks," says Pepe, the young man who cleans the toilets. "The ones with big dicks take hours to wrap the towel around themselves." Some like to pretend that they're not here for sex. "That queen," continues Pepe, "pretends to be an executive. He takes a magazine and starts to read outside the steam bath, like he was at a business meeting."

The Latin sauna lacks the honesty of the North American saunas. Despite the fact that it is a place for sex, it pretends not to be, as though people are just there for the sake of being there. "And why are you here?" Pepe asks. "To do a study on saunas," I reply. "Oh yeah? Then I'm Oprah," he answers sarcastically. "Oh, I see you have a pen in your hand." Pepe says goodbye and begins to clean the floor.

There is a small sauna room, a TV room with old furniture, four showers, two toilets, and two small rooms where couples can have sex. Each of these rooms contains a metal-framed bed with a vinyl-covered mattress. There is no electric light. "The vinyl is a real problem," says Claudio, a twenty-one-year-old client. "You sweat like a pig and it sticks to your back and feels horrible."

In another small room, massages are given by a masseur who is generally a *cachero*. The door is closed, indicating that a client is inside. Genaro, a young man of about twenty, tells us that a hair stylist is inside with David, the most well-endowed masseur in the place. "How do you know he's a hair stylist?" we ask with some curiosity. "The queen goes in with a brush and hair spray to fix her hair and go to work. She had a transplant and needs to cover the holes they made in front. When her hair gets messed up she looks like a broken doll," he tells us with total confidence.

The place is dirty and cockroaches can be seen wandering freely from the sauna room. "When there's nothing to do we entertain ourselves by killing roaches," says Claudio. "Once I thought a man was caressing my back and it was a miserable, fat black cockroach, a bug that you can't even squash because it stinks like hell." "Doesn't it disgust you to have sex with so many bugs around?" we ask. "Actually, it turns me on when a place is full of animals. I feel like Jungle Jane."

There is not a single information poster about AIDS in the establishment, despite the fact that the owner attended a prevention course. "I can't put posters in here—people would worry. They come here to have fun and relax and not think about bad things," he adds. "But don't you think it's in your interest that people don't get infected, so that you don't lose your clients?" we ask. "Well, there will always be more queens in this country. You know, they breed like rabbits here and every week there's thousands of new ones."

The other sauna is called Jolon. It is also located in downtown San José, on the second floor of an old building. A large sign above the entrance bears the name of the place without indicating that it is a sauna, to discourage visits from people who are not homosexuals. It is open from 2 to 9 p.m.

Clients must ring a bell as they climb the stairs so that the attendant will open the metal gate. An entrance fee of 300 colones is charged and visitors receive a blanket, a towel, and a key to their respective locker. Then another locked door leading into the sauna is opened. Next to it is an office belonging to a woman lawyer. Sometimes, her clients and those from the sauna run into each other on the stairs. "One day I was walking upstairs and who should I meet but my aunt going to the lawyer's office," recalls Joaquín, a client. "I nearly died, because the old broad is such a gossip." "What did you do?" we ask. "I went into the lawyer's office so she wouldn't realize I was going to the sauna. I had to pay for an appointment for nothing and ended up without any money!"

The sauna has a large bar with a television, where pornographic videos are shown every day. There is another room with a TV showing regular programs. Here, there are no chairs, only three foam mattresses covered with vinyl on the floor. There are also four smaller rooms with just enough space for a mattress on the floor. This where the more private sexual encounters take place.

This sauna is in better shape than the first. It is cleaner and has two showers with no partition between them. The only toilet in the establishment bears a Ministry of Health poster which reads "Safe Sex: Just one healthy sexual partner."

Like the other two establishments, the Laton Sauna is located in the center of San José. The notice by the entrance says "Gymnasium." At one time there was very little traffic on the street where it is located, but now there is a bus stop, which has become a problem for some clients who are afraid that they might be seen entering.

To enter through the main door, clients must ring a bell, and José, the administrator, opens the metal gate. José decides who will be admitted. He will not open the door to people who are unknown or unattractive. "No sir," he says to an older man, "this gymnasium is only for young people. You should find one for older people." "But there aren't any gyms for older people, kid. Anyhow, this is not a gym," says the man indignantly. "Well, you're no bodybuilder either!" replies José.

Half an hour later, José makes an exception to the rules. This time the prospective clients happen to be six players from a Dutch soccer team that is visiting the country. "Welcome to Laton! How can I help you?" says José in good English. "We want sex!" replies one of the players. José is mesmerized by their good looks and virility. "Please, come in, make yourselves at home. Here at Laton it's like being in Amsterdam. We also have high-quality cheese here that will make you feel great." Barely five minutes after the players' arrival, José is already phoning all his clients. "Come over immediately! Some Dutch guys have just arrived and I promised them lots of action." Within a few hours the sauna is full. Word has gotten around San José that a bunch of tall, blond, well-built soccer players have arrived at Laton's. More than fifty clients show up that day. "But why are you charging more today?" a regular client complains. "Well, because today we're offering imported meat and Dutch milk," replies José.

Clients leave their valuables in a sealed bag that is kept at the front desk and receive a locker key, a bar of soap, a towel, and a blanket. Unlike the other saunas, the towels here are very short. "This little towel is no good, my balls hang out," a client complains. "Look, Luis, hold your gut in and stop whining," chides José. "Anyway, that way you'll fool the clients with those huge balls. They'll think the rest of the goods are the same size."

The sauna has a very large bar with a TV that shows pornographic videos on Fridays. Next to the bar is a dark room that the manager calls the "music room." I go into the room and see three people masturbating. I leave and walk over to watch the movie that is being shown. Two super-macho Americans are in full action. "I don't know why José shows these movies. We never get men with dicks that size here," remarks Gerardo, a twenty-six-year-old client who watches the movie with indifference. "Shut up!" says Juan, a man of about forty. "Did you see the Dutch soccer players who arrived?" He has hardly finished talking when the other man has already disappeared.

The establishment has two sauna rooms: a large one and a small one with capacity for three people. Both are dimly lit and are also used for sexual encounters. The clients are gathered in the large room where the Dutchmen are. When things heat up, the footballers take off their towels and show off their wares. Three clients approach them and do the same. They are all naked. Looks become more penetrating and passion becomes evident. One of the clients who can no longer stand the heat pretends to complain and leaves, saying, "I'm fed up with underdevelopment. The Europeans outstrip us even with the size of their dicks. How humiliating!"

There is a TV room with vinyl-covered mattresses, two toilets, and two showers. Both toilets have Ministry of Health posters about AIDS. A staircase leads to the second floor where the lockers are kept. Another staircase leads to the "gym," which contains a few weight training machines that have seen better days. The machines are there to convince the authorities that this is a gym. Carlos describes an official visit:

> One day the Health Ministry raided this place and the guys who sweep and clean the bathrooms moved the machines and began to exercise to make them think that they were in a gym. Even the administrator, who's the laziest bum and hates to exercise, began to lift weights. The poor guy couldn't sit down for a week! Anyhow, the health officials knew it was all a cover-up. When they left they told José that the only muscle he'd developed was his sphincter.

Next to this gym are two small rooms. A notice on one of them says "Storeroom," though the room is used for sex. The other room has no door. Each has a vinyl-covered mattress on the floor. One of the sauna's regular clients tells us that even marriages—albeit very fleeting ones—have taken place behind its walls:

> One day I met a handsome, masculine peasant guy who was real hot in the sauna. We went into that room and had fantastic sex. I honestly felt that I had found the man of my life. The guy knew how to make love, but he also knew how to make you feel loved. Our relationship was alternately tender and passionate when it needed to be. He told me it had been the best fuck of his life and that he could never leave me. I agreed totally. There was such a mysterious chemistry between us that I felt that this man had to be mine. I accepted an invitation to dine after we had bathed. I went into the shower and dreamed about leaving the sauna and taking this macho guy home. When I returned to the room I noticed he wasn't there and thought he was taking a shower. I waited for him with the longing of true love. As I waited, I heard a couple going into the next cubicle. Soon you could hear moans of ecstasy. As there was still no sign of my macho man, I took a peek through a small hole. And who should I see? My great love, but this time he was being possessed by another!

Unlike the previous two saunas, this one charges clients 350 colones as they leave.

In our 1989 survey of men who frequent gay bars, 24 percent admitted to having visited saunas and having spent an average of two hours a week there.[2] On this occasion, we did not ask questions about visits to other public places. Our ethnographic observations showed that a few hundred gay men frequented parks, public toilets, and movie theaters. On an average day, the ethnographer reported the number of clients as follows:

Parque Monumental	43
Alleyways	18
Toilets	46
Derelict house	12
Movie theaters	50
Sauna Laton	32
Sauna Decoro	18
Sauna Jolon	28
Total	247

On a busy day, the figures were as follows:

Parque Monumental	78
Alleyways	34
Toilets	66
Derelict house	31
Movie theaters	129
Sauna Laton	70
Sauna Decoro	78
Sauna Jolon	48
Total	534

In 1990, these were the most important public sex places in San José. There were other less frequented places, which were not studied: the toilets at the main universities and La Llanura park, where there was only limited sexual activity at that time. One or two movie theaters also showed some activity. However, the above were the main PSPs. By 1998, as we shall see, the situation had changed dramatically.

Chapter 3

The Geography of Desire: 1998

Public sex has undergone a significant development in the past eight years, both in terms of the number and diversity of the participants and their sexual practices. In 1990, only the clients of the Beirut movie theater were divided up according to specific sexual preferences. Now, all the PSPs are divided into areas to cater to different sexual tastes. The purpose of this specialization is to reduce the time needed to make sexual contacts and to make it easier. In a globalized world, where time gets shorter, it makes sense for prostitutes to divide up the different benches or spaces among heterosexuals, gays, Nicaraguans, those who are active, and those who are passive. In this way, clients can more easily select their merchandise. Integrated markets and the collapse of tariff barriers have finally reached the underdeveloped nations. One of the "Chicago boys"* is now director of the Central Bank and in the Parque Principal, penises are exhibited according to size.

PARQUE MONUMENTAL

This is the only park in the capital that has not been remodeled or rebuilt in recent years. Public telephones have been installed on the north and south sides of the park, and there are also bus stops and taxi stands on the north side. The most remarkable thing about the place is that it is still unlit. Although the alleyway is still used, the derelict house has been demolished and turned into a private parking lot.

* "Chicago boys" is a term for economists associated with Milton Friedman and the University of Chicago's conservative fiscal policies in Latin America.

One of the main changes that have taken place is that contacts now occur throughout the day. Another is that the park has become specialized. The south and west sides of the park are frequented by sex workers, whose ages range from approximately seventeen to twenty-five, and who offer their services at night. They position themselves strategically, according to their sexual orientation: those in the southeastern sector are predominantly gays who work as prostitutes, while those in the southwestern sector are bisexual or heterosexual prostitutes.

Another specific group that frequents the park are the locusts, young criminals and muggers who, among other things, make money from gay sex. These young street kids rob gays and sex workers alike. However, as we shall see, the division between mugger and sex worker is sometimes nonexistent.

One of the points of greatest attraction is the metal gazebo located in the center of the park, and the trees around it. This is the scene of what is termed a "ballet": male group sex. We see a young man of about twenty-one take out his penis and begin to masturbate. About twenty men, participants and spectators, take part in the orgy. Another change has been the generalization of micturition. Urinating or pretending to do so is now a group affair. Occasionally, you can see up to ten men pretending to urinate, a phenomenon seldom seen before.

Prostitution has also become more common and more open. Given that sex workers have their own space, clients do not need to waste time trying to decipher who is who. They approach in their cars and after inspecting the available "goods," they make contact with the prostitutes. The average fee is between 3,000 and 5,000 colones ($12 and $18), depending on whether or not they agree to penetrate or be penetrated.

Public phones have become instruments of public sex. Clients have memorized phone numbers and often make calls to pick up contacts or to have phone sex. The ethnographer recorded one of the calls he received.

> Hello, who's calling?
> Armando, at your service.
> Do you really want to serve me? I've got a real hard-on.

That's great, but I'm doing a study on public sex.
Quit fooling! Can you describe yourself?
Well, I'm twenty-three, tall, not too heavy, black hair . . .
And what's it look like?
What does what look like?
Your dick.
It's where it should be, unless it's dropped.
Are you going to fool around, or are you going to be serious?
I just want to ask a few things, that's all. I'll tell you about my dick if you answer some questions.
Like what? [the voice sounds irritated]
How many times a week do you call this number?
I call every night.
And you always have phone sex?
Yes. Sometimes I meet people and we go someplace else.
How long have you been making calls here?
About two years. It's very exciting. Well, are you going to tell me what it's like?
My dick is very small, barely the size of a finger.
[The call ends abruptly as the caller slams the phone down.]

The alleyway, meanwhile, continues in full swing. The number of participants has increased both in the park and in the alley.

NEW PICKUP PARKS

Public sex has gradually spread to other public parks in San José. Right in the heart of the city is the Parque Principal (Main Park), the most important park in the capital. Located in front of a church, it covers about an acre of land and was recently restored as part of the city council's urban renewal program.

Contacts here are primarily between sex workers and their clients, though it is well known that the area around a nearby fast-food restaurant is a social meeting place for gays, especially young ones.

The area where the public phones are located, to the west of the square, is an important pickup point. People pretend to call and begin to exchange glances either with other callers or with those who stand in line pretending to wait to make a call. "You know I have a real hard-on" a young man is saying on the phone, "and there's a guy who's waiting to make a call." This is a way of coming on to the guy who is waiting. We notice how, when he hangs up and leaves, the man who was pretending to wait in line to make a call follows him and they make contact.

Special mention should be made of the public toilets in the fast-food restaurant located just north of Parque Principal, where sexual encounters that have begun in the park are continued. The rest rooms are located at the far end of the restaurant, which itself is a meeting place for the city's gay community. The toilets offer a measure of privacy. One of the ethnographers witnessed a sexual encounter there. As he entered, he saw several individuals gathered around the washbasins and at the urinals by the wall. One of them, standing at the urinal, was showing his penis to a young man beside him, who proceeded to masturbate him. Though they appeared anxious at the possible arrival of a security guard, the presence of the ethnographer did not bother them in the least. Such encounters appear to be fairly common here.

To the west of Parque Principal is another square with similar characteristics, the Parque de La Misericordia. Located in front of the church after which it is named, this park has also been remodeled as part of the urban renewal plan, and has a structure similar to the previous park, though this place is much better maintained and cleaner than the first. It is also less crowded.

Here, sex workers of Nicaraguan origin are the absolute majority. The process of making contacts is the same as in the Parque Principal, but here the sex workers usually sit on the many benches around La Misericordia, where clients seek them out.

Just north of downtown San José are two other parks that form part of this geography of desire: Colombia Park and Pinochet Park.

Both are located in one of the capital's most conservative and traditional districts, surrounded by buildings of great urban importance. They both contain numerous statues, such as one of La Loba, a female guerrilla fighter and feminist writer who wrote just one extraordinary story: "The Story of a Body Which Never Published."

On the south side of Pinochet Park is Thai Pei, one of the city's main heterosexual brothels. Here there is a constant flow of men—both locals and foreigners—especially at night. During the past two years, Pinochet Park has become a meeting point for female sex workers and their clients, and more recently, transvestite prostitutes have begun to work this area. Both transvestites and prostitutes perform hurried oral sex and masturbation in the surrounding area.

As for Colombia Park, some male sex workers mention it as a pickup point. They usually gather around the edge of the park in the afternoon to wait for clients who arrive by car or on foot.

SHOPPING MALLS

San Jose has recently experienced a boom in the construction of U.S.-style commercial centers or shopping malls. One of the most popular is the Saint Pamela Mall, located at the entrance to the capital's eastern sector.

During the first months after the mall was opened, the public toilets became the preferred places for certain kinds of sexual contacts, especially masturbation and oral sex. For this reason, the management adopted restrictive measures, such as the closure of most of the bathrooms in the side corridors and strict controls in the men's toilets near the eating areas. However, public sex continues in the bathrooms of the mall's movie theaters, mainly after the movies have begun, as is also the case in other commercial centers.

UNIVERSITIES

University campuses have become very popular public sex places, both for heterosexuals and homosexuals. Sexual activity occurs in the toilets of private and public universities at all hours.

The University of the Republic, in San Pablo, is one of the country's leading state universities. Those who come to the campus in search of sex start to arrive around noon, and stay for a few hours. Unlike other places, the action here takes place in broad daylight, for which reason the behavior codes vary considerably. People who frequent the campus for sex usually wear sports clothes or lycra, which allows them to show off their genitals.

Some places are well known as pickup points or to signal availability. One is the public telephone located just outside the School of Geometry (in the northwestern sector of the campus), which the university's own security staff call the "gay phone." This phone rings constantly and if the person who answers is willing, the caller will soon appear. As one of the security guards tells us, this is "telemarketing, because people can do their cruising from home."

Other well-known pickup spots on the university campus are the men's toilets. A visit is enough to see the sexual graffiti and slogans daubed on the walls as well as telephone numbers offering services to show that these places are popular with the university's gay population. This afternoon, however, something unusual is going on. A woman enters the toilets with two men. We follow behind them and as we enter, one of the occupants whispers to us: "Did you see how the broad went into one cubicle and the two guys into another?" Our confidant stands there listening. Moans can be heard coming from both cubicles. "That broad is jerking off listening to the two gays," he tells us. He heads toward her cubicle and says, "Honey, you want some help? Why don't you open the door and I'll keep you company?" The woman does not reply and continues moaning. The young man returns to thc urinal and begins to masturbate. He shouts at the woman, "What a waste, bitch! I have to do it alone!" He looks at us hoping to get our sympathy. When the moans from all four (at very different rhythms) subside, the two gays come out of the cubicle and tell us, "Guys, please leave so our friend can go without being seen." We all leave the toilets.

PUBLIC POOLS

The Balneario del Fuego, a public swimming pool and spa, is the only place on our map of desire that is located outside San José. The place is full of young people, adolescents, and children as well as families and groups of friends, though there are also older people, all of them from the lower social strata.

The spa has become a popular meeting place for some sectors of the gay community, especially on weekdays. The observers were able to identify a number of well-known gays, including a male sex worker who is very popular in the capital's gay bars. Among the information gathered at the spa was the fact that many hairstylists flock to the spa on Mondays, when they normally take the day off work.

One way to exhibit the genitals is by wearing tiny thongs or tight-fitting swimsuits. When two men are attracted to each other, they head for the showers and the dressing rooms. Some men stand guard at the entrance so that others can have sex inside. In the showers, we notice a sex worker soaping himself with his penis totally erect. An effeminate man, a well-known hairdresser, bathes beside him and then makes a sign for him to follow the hairdresser into the dressing room. Both enter while four others help to stand guard as they watch the sexual encounter. Amid all the action, two athletes enter the showers and watch the movement in the changing room from afar. "Don't go near there; they're fucking in there," one of them shouts loudly, so that everyone will hear. More men gather to look.

LA LLANURA

If there is a new, almost mythical place fixed in the minds of nearly the whole gay population of Costa Rica, it is La Llanura park, nicknamed by many La Finca (The Farm), a paradise of anonymous public sex in the country. The area is completely accessible. There are no obstacles around the perimeter to restrict access and it is easy to enter on foot and by car. There are five major entry points for cars and the entire place is crisscrossed by paved roads leading to four large parking areas inside the park. The lighting is conspicuous by its absence.

At night, La Llanura is taken over by men who come in search of sex. The visitors are of every age, from youngsters of eighteen or nineteen to older men age sixty or seventy. They are also of a visibly higher social class than the clients at most other places: many of the clients turn up in expensive new cars (BMWs, Pathfinders, Toyotas).

Those who frequent the place report that sexual activity in La Llanura begins at nightfall. As soon as the sports players have left the soccer and baseball pitches located in the southwestern sector of the park at around 5 or 6 p.m., sexual encounters begin between people who arrive on foot and who use the cover from a dense line of trees to hide from prying eyes.

But it is at night, especially on weekends, when La Llanura—particularly the western sector—becomes The Farm, where men come in search of impersonal sex with other men.

Visitors to La Llanura must become familiar with the behavior code. In the first place, a car is almost indispensable. Clients drive along the streets at low speed with their lights on, while around them other cars circulate in the same way. This is how initial contacts are established.

The next step in the ritual is to facilitate a more direct contact. To do this, the client drives through the car parks to see who is there, or else leaves his own car in one of the parking lots. He immediately turns off his car lights: this is the first sign that he is looking for a sexual contact. Soon one or more cars will approach and do the same thing.

After getting out of their cars, two or three individuals hang around the changing rooms near the soccer pitch. A young man of about twenty is the center of attention for the other two. The car owners approach him. They do not say anything. The young man allows one of them to kiss him passionately. The third man stands behind, rubbing his erect penis against the young man without removing his pants. Then the third man gently takes off the young man's belt and lowers his pants. The man who kisses him finishes taking off his underpants. He caresses his buttocks, grabs him by the waist, and asks him to turn around. As the young man turns, the third man begins to fellate the one who has put on a condom, as if to lubricate it. The young man bends over and the one who was kissing him now begins to penetrate him. By this time, another fifteen cars have parked in the area and a circle of spectators surrounds the two men and the young man. Most of the onlookers masturbate as they watch the spectacle. Then, the man who is penetrating the young man asks him to walk around the circle. Each bystander can touch and kiss either of the two men. The third man ends up performing oral sex on one of the spectators.

PORNOGRAPHIC MOVIE THEATERS

Other new places in this tour of public sex locales are the movie theaters, especially those showing movies which could be classified as pornographic, of which there are several in the capital. Eight years ago, the only movie theater used for public sex was the Beirut, which has now been closed down. However, the movies shown there were not pornographic and the theater did not officially qualify as a sex place. The new movie theaters where public sex occurs do not hide their eroticism. Nor do they discriminate against sexual orientation. Heterosexuals and homosexuals have divided the space between them to have their sexual encounters.

The Limon City movie theater is located in one of the capital's red-light districts, a few blocks south of Second Avenue, and is one of the oldest movie theaters in San José. The building, with its pale blue facade and pink doors, is hardly known for its decorative good taste. The decor is shabby, with large posters of movies that one guesses to be appalling and others of old Mexican porn movies which have probably been stuck to the walls for forty years or more.

The place is unlit, except for four orange lamps inside and the glare from the movie screen itself. A black cube serves as a support for the present projection equipment—a video machine (the movie theater no longer shows movies on film, but videos). On the night of our visit a movie titled *Insatiable* was being shown.

Aficionados of public sex also have Cinema 545 at their disposal, an establishment similar to the previous one but with a few notable differences. Although this theater shows pornographic movies from Europe, especially from Italy (such as *Flamenco Ecstasy,* shown on the night of the observation), is in far better shape than the Limon City. It is clean, well managed, and tickets cost 700 colones.

Unlike the Limon City, this movie house shows films. Though the material is equally pornographic, it is of superior quality with better scripts, more attractive actors, and, in general, offers something more than simple, nonsequential sexual encounters.

These theaters are predominantly frequented by men. Among the fifty or so people at the Limon City, there was only one woman accompanied by her partner, while at the Cinema 545 there were three women, all with partners. The average age of the audience was thirty to fifty years, though we also observed a few younger people and some older ones.

The division of the rooms, especially at the Limon City, is accompanied by an extreme polarization in accordance with practices and sexual orientation. The rear right-hand section is where the gays congregate to have different kinds of sex. The rest of the theater, however, is the territory of apparently heterosexual men.

When the movies get "hot," a stream of men head for the toilets. At the Limon City theater there are three stalls with open doors. Men are sitting on the three toilet bowls. Soon others decide to enter. One stops and begins to take off his pants. He takes out his erect penis and looks at someone who is outside the stall. The latter looks at the occupant of the next stall and compares the "goods." The first man has a larger and thicker penis than the second, so he chooses the first stall. He enters and takes down his pants. The man who was waiting for him decides to fellate him. However, they do not close the door. Other clients, including the man in the next stall, watch the scene. The protagonists enjoy the attention. When the man who is being fellated is on the point of ejaculating, he abruptly withdraws his penis and returns to his seat. Half an hour later, he returns to the bathrooms to begin another encounter.

In the Cinema 545, the main activity takes place in the seats. In the darkest area, one of the three women present is being passionately kissed by a man, apparently her boyfriend. However, he leaves her for a few minutes to go to the bathroom. Another man who is sitting two rows behind the woman leaves his seat and sits next to her. The woman looks at him and pretends to be uninterested. Then she turns to look at him and smiles. The man kisses her and puts his hand under her blouse. Since it has buttons down the front, he takes it off completely and also removes her bra. The woman's previous companion returns from the bathroom. Instead of being angry, he sits down without saying a word. While the other man kisses his girlfriend, he opens the man's zipper and takes out his penis. He begins to suck it. A few seconds later, the woman says something that suggests she is going to leave. The man who has been kissing her allows the other man to continue giving him oral sex while she goes to the women's rest room.

PORNOGRAPHIC VIDEOS

Special mention should be made of a pornographic video rental business that also doubles as a public sex place. Video Pop, as the place is called, is located in the heart of the capital, in an old house painted in loud colors (yellow and orange) with a large sign bearing its name. It is located in an area frequented by prostitutes, where there are many office and apartment buildings and large numbers of cars circulate.

Video Pop began by renting pornographic videos and eventually expanded its services to include video shows, live sex shows, and private areas where different kinds of sexual activities are available. The establishment has many plastic seats and benches where clients sit. The main feature of this old house is that it constantly appears to be in the process of being remodeled and always looks half-finished; ever since it opened, it has had unpainted walls, wooden divisions, and unfinished floors. In general terms, it is a dirty place.

Video Pop opens at 2 p.m. and closes at 11 p.m., and its services are divided according to the population: homosexual or heterosexual. Video rentals cost 500 colones for heterosexuals and double for homosexuals. The owner justifies this difference by saying that gay videos are "harder to come by and many clients steal them." The cost of watching a video on the premises, without renting it, is also 500 colones.

On entering, clients are greeted by the owner at the reception desk. Beyond is a large room containing a video collection from which clients can make a selection. Along the corridor are two viewing rooms: one, a small room with a large TV, a videocassette machine, and chairs, is for gays. Next to it is a dark room where all kinds of sexual activities take place and a small room that is used by a female prostitute to have sex with nongay men. The larger room shows heterosexual videos and has a bathroom at the far end.

We walk into the room for gays. About fifteen young men ages eighteen to twenty-five are watching a porn movie. The owner walks in every so often, using sexual language to "warm up" the clients. "Okay, okay, let's get our pants off; I want to see some dicks," he tells the clients. Some giggle nervously and don't know what to do. "Anyone who won't show me his dick, I'll take him to the whore in the straights' room," he says, pretending to be angry. "Come on, Carlos, I know you like people to see your hard-on. Take your pants down." The owner is heterosexual but he knows that the sooner his clients lose their inhibitions, the sooner others can come in and pay to watch. Only the young man called Carlos dares to take his pants down. The owner turns to an effeminate young kid, who looks around with frightened eyes. "You, come here! Don't tell me that you don't want all of this up inside you," he says as he pulls the boy out of his chair by the hand. "I decide what everyone does here, 'cause you can't fool me," says the owner, smiling. He hands a condom to Carlos. The young men laugh. "You, come here and suck him—he's got a good tool," the owner tells a young man who appears to be a student, and who, surprisingly, obeys him. He pushes three others who do not want to join in toward a curtain that separates the heterosexual area, to "warm up by watching," as he says. In this room, a female prostitute is having sex with four men who take turns penetrating her. After watching for a while, the three young men return to the gay room and begin to masturbate. The owner encourages them. "Come on, boys! Don't be shy; don't be discouraged—just remember to wear a condom."

SAUNAS

The same saunas continue to operate as in previous years. But the number of clients and the prices have increased. Currently, the entrance fees range from 1,100 to 1,300 colones ($5 to $6). However, the most striking change has been the specialization of these establishments and the opening of new saunas.

One of these is called Adonis. It is located on the top floor of a narrow building, and to enter clients ring a bell on a black door leading to some stairs. At the end is an electric gate that is opened from inside. The hours of operation are similar to the other saunas, from 2 to 10 p.m. Liquor, beer, and soft drinks are sold on the premises, though there is no refrigerator to keep them cold. There is only a small icebox whose contents are quickly sold and must be replenished from a nearby store.

Adonis is the only sauna where sex does not take place among the clients, but rather with sex workers who are employed as masseurs. The masseurs gather in the sauna's TV room, wearing short, tight-fitting lycra pants, swimsuits, or underpants. One of them, the most popular with clients, is a young man measuring almost 5′ 11″ tall, dark-skinned, with well-defined muscles and very well-endowed genitals. "How much do you charge?" we ask. "Depends on what we do," he answers. "If you want me to stick it up you, it costs 7,000 colones, and with a condom. I don't make exceptions. Three thousand for a rub." "Why do you charge so much?" we ask. "Well, just imagine this all stiff," he says, showing me his penis.

NUMBERS

Not only have public sex places diversified and specialized, but the number of clients has doubled. On an average day, nearly 600 people have sex and on the busiest days more than 1,000:

Place	Minimum	Maximum
Parque Monumental	80	150
Alleyway	40	80
Parque Principal	60	90
Restaurant toilets	30	50
Misericordia Park	40	80
Parque Colombia	20	40
Parque Pinochet	20	40
La Llanura Park	45	300
Limon City	30	60
Cinema 545	25	50
Sauna Laton	30	70
Sauna Decoro	20	50
Sauna Jolon	30	60
Sauna Adonis	30	60
Balneario del Fuego Spa	30	50
University of the Republic	25	50
Malls	15	30
Video Pop	40	80
Total	610	1,330

Chapter 4

Man . . . Without Words

In the beginning was the Word; and the Word was with God, and the Word was God. (John: 1:1)

The places described in the previous chapters are characterized by the absence of words. Whether heterosexual or homosexual, people use few words. When they talk, it is about inconsequential things. None of the conversations has anything to do with what is actually happening. One man talks about the weather. Another asks what the time is. A third asks for a match.

The fact that no words are exchanged does not mean that the communication is more or less intimate, or that people are more or less interested in others. For Derrida, traditional Western thinking has focused on the superiority of the spoken over the written word. This is what he called "logocentrism," or the idea that truth is closer to the spoken word.[1] Moreover, our Western thinking has also been influenced by what he called the "metaphysics of presence." This means that we believe we are closer to the truth when people talk to each other and directly express what they think. One only writes when one is not present, and this can lead to mistakes. Written language is thus seen as the "great absence" and as a simple and imperfect substitute for oral language.

Our culture teaches us that to have sexual relations we must first know the other person. "Know" means "talk to." If we do not talk, we do not know someone, and therefore our conduct is considered immoral. Thus, Hollywood has accustomed us to having to listen to a series of stupid dialogues before presenting us with the first sex scene. When things do not happen that way, as in the movie *Fatal Attraction*, people will pay for rushing into sex. But if we were to pay close attention to the verbiage uttered by actors before they remove their clothes, we would notice that they use metaphors to communicate. "You've broken my heart," says an actress. Nobody whose heart has literally been broken could continue acting. This is another example of the fact that we say things which, although they may come out of our own mouths, actually come from fiction, from books—in short, from the written word.

If people go to a public place to have sex, we think they are promiscuous and vulgar because they do not "really" know their sexual partners. However, the same philosopher shows us that this hypothesis is false. Derrida does not believe any real difference exists between what is written and spoken, between what is present and what is absent. We do not get to know people better because they express their thoughts directly or because they do so in a letter, a poem, or a movie script. We all use a language that is predetermined by what is written. We do not know one another more or better because we speak or because we touch. We might instead conclude that we get to know a person who represents to us a script of his or her innermost desires more intimately than another who talks to us like a parrot. To illustrate this, let us do a visualization with our eyes shut (ask someone to read the following to you):

> Imagine that you are in the public park of your fantasies. Someone you find attractive approaches you. He looks into your eyes and, without saying anything, asks you to reveal to him a sexual fantasy, a story which Judeo-Christian thought has made you feel is shameful and which you have not told anyone. You resist at first, but then you focus on this person and think that he would be the ideal person to realize this fantasy. You like him. He is like the model you have pursued since childhood. Your hormones are stirred up. You try to flee and begin to walk away. However, your feet feel heavy. Your body does not want to leave. The person follows you patiently and again looks into your eyes. "Why fight this desire?" you think. Yes, you decide to reveal your fantasy. But it cannot be done with words. You must invent a language to communicate it to him. Nobody else will know about it. In a few minutes,

> you are doing it. Is this person a stranger? Does he know something that no one else suspects?

Is this intimate or not?

THE LANGUAGE OF METAPHOR

Let us remember that a metaphor is a word used to refer to another which it substitutes for, suggesting a similarity between the two. When someone in the park tells us, "This is a pickup place," he is using the language of metaphor, the language of literature and fiction. Although the informer is present, he is using the language of literature and to understand it, we must find its meaning in a dictionary or in the written words of a novel.

Public sex places prioritize what we term nonverbal messages. However, just because words are not used, we should not conclude that there is no language. In public sex places, the body is the paper on which words are written. The organs are laden with meaning and their manipulation provides us with the narrative.

When we talk with someone, we are not able to go beyond the discourses that have been learned or read elsewhere. "I believe in love and I think you're the light of my life," a suitor once told me in a bar. "Does he think my face looks like a flashlight, or what?" I thought to myself. "I probably have a greasy face and it's very shiny." To understand this lovely, corny metaphor, I would have had to read about the Cathars and their ideas that we are bodies which enclose the divine light. Did I get to know that romantic individual any better because he uttered that corny literary cliché or would it have been better to know him in a park, performing the role of a sexual fantasy, also taken from a literary work? For now, guided by our informers, we shall give one of the many interpretations of the language of public places.

From about 4:00 in the afternoon, heterosexual couples begin to arrive at the Parque Monumental and sit down on the benches, especially those where there is less light. Here they spend many hours talking, kissing, and, when possible, masturbating each other. The park, then, is not just a center for homosexual activity, but also for heterosexual activity.

Julio, a sex worker who is a regular at this park, describes some of the heterosexual couples who meet regularly each week. For example, Armando, a friend of Julio, is a twenty-two-year-old medical student at the university. He looks a little older than his age and is quite attractive. Celina, his girlfriend, is a sixteen-year-old high school student who lives in an eastern district of the city. Armando waits for her at 6:30 p.m. every Monday to walk her to the bus. They sit on a bench and gaze into each other's eyes. "Both know that she has to be home at 7:30 for dinner. Her parents are very strict and they don't allow her to have a boyfriend," explains Julio.

As on any other Monday, the sweethearts sit on a bench on the southern side of the park. They begin to kiss passionately. From a distance, we can see the young man placing his hand under the girl's skirt. We could surmise that he touches her intimate parts but it is not really clear, since he makes sure that her skirt covers his hand. She holds his hand and gently takes it out. The hand under her skirt could mean that today he wants to have sex. The hand outside would imply that she does not want to yet or that she does not want to be considered easy, or that perhaps she doesn't want to today but another day, when she feels more like it, she might. Derrida would say that it is impossible to determine the infinite number of possibilities; in other words, it is "undeterminable."

Julio points to another couple two benches farther on. "She's an old broad who works at the government building nearby." She comes to the park and meets a guy who works at the hospital. The woman takes out a small white cloth from her purse. When this comes out, the man unzips his fly. It seems that the small white cloth means that his sexual organ can come out of its "casing." He touches her breasts and she begins to masturbate him, covering his penis with the white cloth. They do not say a word to each other. His hand on her breasts is a signal that she can grab his penis and rub it. When he finishes, she gathers up her little white cloth, folds it, and puts it back in her purse. The semen in her purse seems to imply that the sexual encounter is over. Is this an illicit affair? It would appear so, because a few minutes later another man collects the woman in his car. The hospital worker returns to work without even looking at her. You might think that the cloth in the purse is a metaphor to tell us of a relationship that must remain hidden, illicit.

So much so that Julio himself understands it. "When I see either one of them in the street, I pretend not to recognize them; I pretend I've never seen them in the park."

"The most daring couple is the one that sits over there on that bench," says our informer. Come here Wednesday at eight at night you'll see!" We meet Julio at exactly five minutes to eight on Wednesday. A couple of minutes later, a woman of around forty and a young man of eighteen meet at the bench. They arrive separately. They sit down, barely greeting each other. The woman looks like an office worker or a secretary. She takes out a blanket with colored squares and places it over the young man's lap. The blanket suggests that something important is about to happen. The young man moves around beneath the blanket, apparently to remove his belt and take down his pants. Once he stops moving, she understands that he is ready. The woman kneels down and dives under the blanket. "She must give one hell of a great blow job," says Julio.

Heterosexual couples come to do the same as the homosexual ones. However, Julio himself correctly interprets their different metaphors: "Heterosexuals fuck with rags on their laps." This means that somewhere they learned that genitals should not be exposed, even if you have public sex. Penises, breasts, and vulvas are covered with skirts, little white cloths, or colored blankets. This language is very different from the gays'. "The gays go around with their dicks, their asses, and their balls hanging out. The more dicks out in the open air, and the bigger they are, the more they enjoy it. When they want to have sex, they show all they've got," says our interviewee. Moreover, heterosexuals do not display sizes or organs.

Though the couples are present in body, the same cannot be said of language. To understand this, we must follow Julio's example and learn the code as we would any foreign language. However, we would not find a dictionary to explain the meaning of a cloth in a purse, or a colored blanket on someone's lap.

After about 10:00 at night, the heterosexual couples leave the park and the place becomes a gay meeting area. A nonverbal code initiates contact. When two gays meet, one way of showing interest in having sex is to touch their own genitals on the outside of their pants. This gesture is characteristic of many heterosexual men in the country, who generally do it as a sign of manhood. However, in the case of gay men in a public sex place, it has a different connotation. The message here might be: "All this could be yours" or "I want you to touch me and to touch you" or "Look what a great thing I have here for you; it hardly fits in my hand."

Novices soon learn the code, though some interviewees told the ethnographer that at first they did not understand the significance of this gesture. One, Gerardo, recounted the following story:

> To me it's normal to see macho men doing that at any time of the day, and I didn't understand that things are different here. My friends who are experts at picking up contacts here told me that when someone does that in front of you, then you have to do the same. It's the way of answering, "I'm interested too," without having to speak. It's very comfortable and also very exciting.

Another sign for making contact is for a man to walk around jangling a bunch of keys in his hand. This means, "I have a place where we can be together" or "I have a car." Once eye contact has been made with the desired person and the routine questions have been asked (What's your job? Do you live alone or with your family? Where do you live?), he studies the person's character. Attention is paid to his accent, the way he speaks Spanish, and any nervousness or sign of anger in his answers. If, after this "reading," the man concludes that there is no danger, he establishes contact and looks for a darker place. According to Mario, "In the darkest area of the gazebo guys sit down on benches to touch each other and turn each other on. The ones who sit in there are only interested in receiving oral sex. Sitting with your legs apart means "I'm not moving from here. If you want something, you'll have to bend over."

Another common way of making contact, according to Gerardo, is to arrive in a car. Drivers cruise around the park at low speed. Some park on the west or south sides and remain in the car, waiting for someone to come over and talk to them, or they get out of the car for "an inspection tour," as a walk around the park is called.

Pedro explains:

> Guys in cars regularly pass through the park and sometimes fancy vehicles turn around and stop. Someone will get into the car and make the contact. Others park on the west side of the park and wait for someone to pass or for someone to go over and talk to them.

A car stopped at a park means that a private space is available. Once the driver and the walker make contact, the latter gets into the car. Sometimes they masturbate and have oral sex there right away, though they usually go to a place farther away to have sex and then return to the park where the initial contact was made. The way of making contact in the alleyway is slightly different. In the first place, many of the couples who meet in the park end up having sex in this street, so contacts here are more direct and there is less courtship than in the park.

The public toilet is another place that facilitates very direct sexual contact because its small size means that men are confined within a very limited space and performing a physiological task that requires them to touch themselves. People who use the urinal do not talk to each other. All the action takes place very quickly. If a man urinates, it means that he is not interested in the other person. If he doesn't urinate, it means he is. Because there is always the possibility that a heterosexual or a policeman might come in, speed is the name of the game. Part of the excitement of the place is the sense of the forbidden, of something fleeting. "There's no need for long conversations and fastidious courtships," as Mario says.

During different observations conducted from a point near the site, it was possible to see men arriving in cars and parking them in front of the toilets. They would get out of the cars, go inside the toilets, have sex, return to their cars, and leave. Others would park their cars, go to the toilet, contact someone who interested them, return with their contact, and the two would drive off.

Many people visit all three places. Some men begin touring the three places around nine at night and are there until 1:00 or even 3:00 in the morning. The number of people increases on weekends, though during the rest of the week there are always men wandering around the area.

Although the rules of contact in the movie theaters do not vary significantly, the fact that there are different areas of action means that each one functions differently. In the public toilets, for example, sex takes place hurriedly, as in the urinal. Availability is expressed with an exposed penis. In the darker sectors, men can perform acts that are more in line with those of the alleyway, and the seats in certain areas of the theater may be used for courtship, conversation, and an invitation to go to a motel. However, the initial language is nonverbal. If you are interested in a man, you sit next to him and stare at him intently. "That means 'I like you and I want to be with you'," explains Victor. If the person agrees, he remains in his seat.

This is how a regular client describes the scene:

> People come and go, walk downstairs, and wander about all over the place. You can't watch the movie in peace. If someone who isn't part of the scene were to come in here and sit down to watch a movie, they wouldn't be able to see anything because of all the people going back and forth. Sitting next to someone and staring at them is a sign of interest. If you don't want to have sex with the person who sat beside you, then you move.

There are many ways of making contacts. In the seats downstairs, older men directly offer money to anyone willing to go with them to a nearby hotel. In fact, sitting here means that one is looking for a male prostitute. An older man sitting next to a young man means that sex is paid for. "The older man just needs to touch the genitals of the young man to show that he's interested," explains our informant. The prostitute states his price and says little else. If the client gets up and waits for the young man to do the same, it shows that they have an agreement. If the price seems too high, the client remains seated and begins watching the movie again. "This means he's not interested in the deal," says Victor. If that's the case, the young guy will look for another older man and sit beside him.

In the toilet, all a man has to do is enter and other men will approach and touch his genitals without saying a word. In the back of the theater, the more attractive men wait for others to approach them to initiate a sexual contact. Sitting at the back means, "I'm so cute that I don't need to look for anyone. If you want something good, you do the work." Once again, verbal communication is minimal. Upstairs, where the orgies take place, all one needs to do is to join them. However, not everyone is welcome. If three men, for example, are having sex and a fourth tries to join in and is not wanted by any one of them, then the three move somewhere else. "This means that they're not interested in more people," says Victor.

Saunas provide more opportunities for conversation. A man can talk to another man at the bar and then take him to a private room. There is also the option of entering the sauna room and waiting, as is the case in Decoro, for the lights to be turned off, and then approach and touch the person who is next to him, without saying a word. The way to assent is to remove the towel. "This means 'I'm at your disposal'," Pedro explains.

Another way of making contact is to enter one of the rooms, leave the door half open to signal availability, and wait for someone. If someone comes into the cubicle and is not attractive to the person who is there, he gestures "no" with his hand. "If the person lies down with his backside facing outward, it means he's passive in anal sex and that anyone who is active is welcome," adds Pedro.

The language of public places is so complex that anyone can make a mistake. Alvaro, a new client, tells us about his experience:

> The first time I came to the park I didn't know what all these codes meant. I was walking along one of the paths and met this guy who was touching his genitals and looking at me. "How dirty," I thought to myself. "He's probably itching because he's full of lice." I continued walking and another guy did exactly the same. "Oh no! All these guys are infested with lice," I thought, and I decided to run away.

Alberto, a twenty-three-year-old, made a similar mistake in a sauna:

> I've always wanted to help my friends. Because I was the eldest of my brothers and sisters, I always had to cover them up when they were asleep and make sure that they weren't cold. The first time I went to Decoro I noticed that there were two cubicles with the doors open and two guys were asleep on their backs, naked. I felt so sorry for them that I decided to go

in and cover them up with a sheet and close the door, so they wouldn't get a blast of wind. What I got was a blast of his anger! "What's the matter, you crazy shit?" one of them yelled. "D'you think you're the Nanny? Go cover up your grandmother's ass!"

SCHOOL FOR PUBLIC SEX

How is practice determined in a place where sex must be done quickly and verbal language is absent? In heterosexual relations the "scripts" have always been clear because penetration is the man's prerogative. But what happens with anal sex and oral sex between men? How does one decide, in a matter of seconds, who does what to whom? Before public sex places became popular, these decisions were made on the basis of social class. In Latin America, the poor have always been at the social, economic, and sexual service of the rich.

But the class factor is irrelevant in most public places. Because of the danger of robbery, wealth cannot be made visible and clothing is useless to determine it. Education is hard to see in the absence of a spoken language. Thus, the more established criteria that traditionally governed relationships between Latin gays no longer operate. In other words, here money does not determine practice, nor does it serve to teach each person his function. Perhaps the only exceptions to this rule are those drivers who can impress with their cars. But they are a minority.

A more convenient language for these places is the language of North American pornography. The main rules are size, beauty, and youth, which easily allow for the establishment of clear hierarchies in public sex. At the same time, pornography itself not only serves as a language but also as a teacher. After watching so many of these movies, people gradually assimilate their values. Soon, something that was once considered disgusting, such as oral sex, becomes a preferred practice.

Both in pornography and in public sex places, the size of the penis is now the main criterion to establish penetration. Fifteen years ago it was considered vulgar or ridiculous to show one's genitals as a way of attracting sexual partners. Even in 1989, the penis was exposed in a more subtle way, by holding it inside the pants. Only in the urinals would men pull down their zippers and expose themselves. Now, however, the penis is out. In the park, men walk around with erections.

Why the need to expose it? Because size determines function. Those with large penises are the ones who will receive oral or anal "services." No other criterion is needed for two men to reach a quick agreement. "When I take out my dick and compare it and see that it's bigger than my date's, he knows he has to suck me or give me his ass," says Julio. "But what happens if the guy is older than you or seems more educated?" we ask. "Nothing happens. It's the law of the jungle here. If my dick is larger, he either takes it or he looks for another one."

Another criteria is physical attractiveness. As in pornography, the most handsome men receive more attention from the rest. "There's a very good-looking guy who comes here and sits at the back," says Ernesto at the Cinema 545. "The guys take turns to suck him just because he's so gorgeous." When the above criteria are not sufficient, youth serves as a parameter. The youngest men tend to receive oral sex from the older ones, rather than the other way around. "Unless they're prostitutes," says Victor, "the young kids go to the movie houses to find old guys to suck them. If you're getting on in years, your job is to suck," he adds. Humphreys found exactly the same in his study of North American public toilets in the 1960s: "In most cases fellatio is a service performed by an older man upon a younger."[2] After the age of forty, the author found that the practice of passive oral sex was a rarity. Part of aging is losing this privilege.

Although these rules are not universal and are often disregarded, they enable people to reach agreement in a few seconds. It is when these rules are not followed that problems, arguments, and discussions arise.

LANGUAGE AND "LA DIFFÉRANCE"

According to Derrida, the spoken language and words are no less and no more present than a movie script or a García Márquez novel. When we do not know the meaning of a word and look it up in the dictionary, we are given another word for reference. However, we might not know what this one means either, and must continue with our search. Each word of our spoken language is, therefore, referred to another and another ad infinitum. Thus each word when expressed is inhabited by the ghosts of all the words to which it is similar and from which it differs. Derrida termed this "la différance," a very subtle way of telling us that each word needs the other, is "differentiated" from it, and its meaning is postponed or "deferred" by it.

Language is also occupied or inhabited by other languages of reference and of difference. In each one of these, we find another language to which it relates. The language of pornography is no exception: it is permeated by the language of globalization.

The only really important event in this Central American country in the past eight years has been its incorporation into the global market, symbolized by the Internet, where integration also implies specialization. Costa Rica has been forced to leave behind its protectionist policies to compete on an equal footing in the world market. All areas in which the country does not have the competitive advantage because of the small size of its internal market, such as the manufacture of refrigerators, for example, must be abandoned in order to specialize in those where it does have an advantage, such as producing chayotes (a kind of vegetable) or sexual tourism, to cite two examples. The strict laws of supply and demand will determine the criteria and set the guidelines.

As market theory goes, a prostitute with a small penis, for whom there is less demand, will not be able to compete with another who has a large one. "On average, escorts have the larger penis. Otherwise they wouldn't do well in the market."[3] Sooner or later, the sex worker with a smaller organ will adapt to reality: he would do better to mug clients rather than fuck them. Those with more than eight inches, on the other hand, will make more from sex than from robbery. Their organs are like a small business that even allows them to have employees. "My friend has a huge dick and he charges 5,500 colones," says a mugger who operates in the park. "And why the extra 500 colones?" we ask, intrigued by the coefficient. "That's my commission," he replies.

The language of pornography is inhabited by that of University of Chicago economics. Milton Friedman[4] never imagined that when the clients of Costa Rica's public sex places learned the language of public sex from porn movies, they also "imported" his economic theories, which inhabit this language like ghosts. Thus, they not only learned how to suck penises, but also how to set a price for each one. The largest, the prettiest, and the youngest are the most expensive, the most alluring, and the most sought after. In the flesh market, size does matter.

However, as we shall see, the language of pornography, or that of the "Chicago boys," or of postindustrial capitalism, when applied to an underdeveloped country, generates certain tensions. In a Latin American culture obsessed with class differences, in which one sector of the population feels more at home in Miami than in its poorer neighborhoods, the North American pornographic model creates an illusion of democratic capitalism. For a few moments each day, the Nicaraguan mugger, an illegal and dispossessed immigrant who is being sought by immigration agents who want to deport him, becomes, because of the size of his penis, a porno star. His physical attributes bring him respect, admiration, and demand from clients in the park, the movie theater, or the public toilet. Although he may not feel any sexual attraction for these men, he cannot help but feel satisfaction at his popularity and at the high price he commands. The young man feels he has value, that, for an instant, the world has turned upside down, giving him a taste of what things could be like if he had money. Everyone wants to be with him, from the politician who left his car in a nearby parking lot and has removed all distinguishing marks, to the government bureaucrat who has spent the day planning raids on undocumented foreigners.

However, the dream, like every fairy tale, has its end. When the prostitute, like Snow White, finally awakens, he will find a whole bunch of dwarfs that he doesn't want to see. Contrary to what Pat Califia theorizes for the United States,[5] nothing is revolutionary or radical about public sex in Costa Rica. No progress has been made in the revolution against the Judeo-Christian tradition just because people have oral sex in a park, instead of in their bedroom. What is truly revolutionary is that it shows some of its victims that the world could be ordered in a different way. The prostitute who has been aroused from his lethargy by the kiss of a horny prince will never see things in the same way again.

Chapter 5

The Gay Clientele

There is a group that visits public sex places almost daily. It is made up of out-of-the-closet homosexuals who know one another. At any time of night, on any day of the week, regular visitors know they will find someone they have already met.

Other groups do not have social relations with the people who frequent the parks, movie theaters, or public toilets. During the daytime, for instance, it is common to see young university or high school students flocking to the parks to study individually or in groups. Movie theaters have all types of customers, not all of them gay. The same is true of public toilets, university campuses, and recreation centers. Saunas are the only places where these heterosexual groups are absent. At the movie theaters and parks, a few women participate in public sex.

Another group of men who frequent such places are bisexual males, or homosexuals who have not come out and feel they cannot afford to be seen in homosexual bars. Many of these men who are still in the closet are more masculine, less "detectable," which is an added attraction for other gay men.

A key group of regular participants consists of criminals and sex workers; their roles sometimes overlap. Sex workers visit public sex places to find customers and participate in sex acts for money. The intention of the criminals, on the other hand, is to mug their "clients." Police officers also make an appearance from time to time, to repress sexuality, acts of sexual commerce, and crimes. Many of them, as we shall see later, also participate in the sexual life of public places, particularly in parks and university campuses.

THE GAY MODEL OF PUBLIC SEX

As we have seen, gay men who visit bars are one of the groups that participate in public sex. This sector of the homosexual population is the most accessible for quantitative research. The fact that thousands of them visit the dozens of gay bars that pepper San José makes it easy to interview them as part of a survey. Therefore, if one wishes to understand the motivations and expectations of public sex aficionados, they are a key group.

The model of sexuality that is pursued by this group, as we shall soon learn, could be summarized in one phrase: the body and its pleasures. This model has two components: a homosexual identity is in place, and the entire body is involved.

Those who were interviewed did not see their sexuality as merely a form of behavior, but as a way of life. Practically 90 percent of gay men who visit bars define themselves as homosexual or bisexual; there is no difference between those who visit public sex places and those who do not (see Table 5.1). To begin with, they share the belief that people pair off in accordance with the objects of their desire: homosexuals are those who like members of their own sex. Second, they believe that homosexuality is a more or less permanent state of being, something lodged in people's minds. It therefore does not reside in any given part of the body, nor does it exclude any organ; there are no taboo body parts inaccessible to pleasure. Public sex is another way of enjoying the homosexual body. The goal is to stimulate and satisfy all the senses and all the organs.

TABLE 5.1. Sexual Orientation and Attendance at Public Sex Places

Orientation		Visits PSPs	Does not visit PSPs	Total
	(N)	**(164)**	**(137)**	**(301)**
	TOTAL	**100**	**100**	**100**
Homosexual		86.6	85.4	86.0
Bisexual		12.2	10.9	11.6
Heterosexual		1.2	3.6	2.3

According to this model—the body and its pleasures—sexual fantasies are the scripts that allow participants to receive and give the greatest stimuli to the senses. Public places become the stage where fantasies promote the enjoyment of the body.

Most gays who visit bars also visit public places. When asked if they had visited one, 54.5 percent said they had (see Table 5.2). Moreover, as can be seen in Table 5.9, 36 percent visit such places at least once a week, if not more often. The most popular places include saunas (27.6 percent), La Llanura Park (17.9 percent), the Balneario del Fuego Spa (15.6 percent), movie theaters (12.3 percent), the campus of the University of the Republic (11.3 percent), and public toilets (11 percent).

Those who visit such places are mainly young men in search of new experiences. Table 5.3 shows some of their social and demographic characteristics. Most gays who visit public sex places, for instance, are between twenty and twenty-nine years old. However, a third are between thirty and thirty-nine years old.

They are not uneducated, either. On the contrary, most of them have attended university. Unlike the other participants, who have

TABLE 5.2. Visits to Anonymous Public Sex Places, by Place

	(N) (164)
Percentage of respondents who have had sexual relations in a public sex place	54.5
Places visited	
Saunas	27.6
La Llanura Park	17.9
Balneario del Fuego Spa	15.6
Movie theaters	12.3
University of the Republic	11.3
Public toilets	11.0
Alleyways	9.3
Parque Monumental	8.6
Parque Principal	3.0

TABLE 5.3. Sociodemographic Characteristics According to the Practice of Visiting Public Sex Places

	Visits PSPs	Does not visit PSPs	Total
(N)	(164)	(137)	(301)
TOTAL	100	100	100
Age			
• Less than 20	6.7	6.6	6.6
• 20-29	57.3	49.6	53.8
• 30-39	30.5	35.0	32.5
• 40-49	4.9	7.3	6.0
• 50 and older	0.3	1.5	1.0
Studies			
• None	—	—	—
• Did not finish primary school	0.6	1.5	1.0
• Finished primary school	3.1	3.6	3.3
• Did not complete high school	16.0	17.5	16.6
• Completed high school	23.3	17.5	20.6
• Attended university	57.1	59.9	58.2

often had only a few years of schooling, gays are a privileged group. In an underdeveloped country, only a fraction of the population can go to college or to a university. Their motivation for attending public sex places, therefore, has no monetary basis, unlike the other groups in this study.

Users of such facilities are not closet homosexuals. As Table 5.4 shows, they are fairly open about their orientation. When it comes to the awareness their mothers, fathers, and bosses have of their orientation, there are differences. Of those who visit public sex places, 60 percent of their mothers know about their sexual orientation, as opposed to 51 percent among the mothers of those who do not visit public sex places. The same was true of 45 percent of fathers, among those who visit PSPs, and of 30 percent of those who do not. Likewise, 27 percent of the bosses of those who go to PSPs were aware of their employees' orientation while only 32 percent of the bosses of those who do not visit PSPs were equally aware. People who engage in

TABLE 5.4. Known Orientation and Sexual Relationships Depending on Public Sex Place Attendance

	Visits PSPs	Does not visit PSPs	Total
(N)	(164)	(137)	(301)
TOTAL	100	100	100
People who are aware of the respondent's sexual orientation			
Closest heterosexual friend (male)	70.1	70.1	70.1
Closest heterosexual friend (female)	75.0	74.5	74.8
Boss or immediate superior	27.4	32.1	29.6
Father	45.1	30.7	38.5
Mother	60.4	51.8	56.5
Brother(s)	54.6	53.3	53.8
Sister(s)	58.9	53.3	56.1
Wife	3.7	1.5	2.7
Children*	1.8	1.5	1.7
Type of sexual partnership			
Closed	38.4	48.9	43.2
Open	16.5	10.9	14.0
Occasional partners	31.1	13.9	23.3
Celibate with men	11.0	21.9	15.9
Celibate with women	0.6	2.2	1.3
Other	2.4	2.2	2.3

* Significant difference: $\alpha = 5\%$

public sex, then, are more open to other people who play a significant role in their lives. This would undermine the myth that it is men who have not yet come out of the closet who tend to visit such places.

Finally, participants are not loners. It is true that 49 percent claim not to be in a "closed" relationship. However, that still leaves 38 percent who say they are involved in a monogamous relationship, which suggests that their partners are not aware of their illicit sexual escapades.

Table 5.5 shows that the group of men who visit public sex places experienced a somewhat earlier sexual initiation than those who do

TABLE 5.5. Distribution of First Sexual Encounter with a Man, As Related to Habit of Visiting Public Sex Places

	Visits PSPs	Does not visit PSPs	Total
(N)	(164)	(137)	(301)
TOTAL	100	100	100
Age of the respondent at the time of the first sexual encounter			
Under 5	0.6	2.9	1.7
5-9	9.8	10.2	10.0
10-14	28.7	20.4	24.9
15-19	44.4	38.0	41.5
20-24	13.4	16.8	15.0
25 and over	3.0	11.7	7.1
Age of the first sexual partner			
Under 10	4.8	8.0	6.3
10-19	37.5	29.2	33.2
20-29	37.4	43.1	39.9
30-39	16.6	16.1	15.2
40 and older	6.7	3.6	5.3

not. Of those who visit PSPs, 28 percent said they had their first sexual experiences between the ages of ten and fourteen; by contrast, only 20 percent of those who do not visit public sex places made the same claim.

Regarding respondents' regular or occasional sexual partners (see Table 5.6), there are no surprises: those who visit public sex places have more partners than those who do not. Among users, 20 percent say they have had between five and nine sexual partners in the past year; only 5.1 percent of nonusers said the same thing. Three times as many PSP users (8.5 percent) said they have had over ten partners; only 2.9 percent of nonusers made the same claim. In the thirty days prior to being interviewed, 57 percent of those who do not visit public sex places said they had remained celibate; however, only 35 percent of visitors said the same thing. Almost twice as many users (12 percent) as nonusers (6.6 percent) said they have had more than two sexual encounters in the last

TABLE 5.6. Distribution of Variables Related to Regular or Occasional Partners, As Related to Habit of Visiting PSPs

	Visits PSPs	Does not visit PSPs	Total
(N)	(164)	(137)	(301)
TOTAL	100	100	100
Number of regular partners in the past 12 months			
• None	22.6	29.5	25.6
• One	45.1	51.8	48.2
• Two	21.3	11.7	16.9
• Three or more	10.9	18.2	9.3
Average number of regular partners, past 12 months[a,c]	1.3	1.0	1.2
Number of occasional partners, past 12 months[b,c]			
• None	25.6	54.0	38.5
• Fewer than 5	45.7	38.0	42.2
• 5-9	20.1	5.1	13.3
• 10 or more	8.5	2.9	6.0
Average number of occasional partners, past 12 months	1.2	0.5	0.9
Number of sexual contacts, past 30 days			
• None	35.4	57.7	45.5
• One	45.7	33.6	40.2
• Two	12.2	6.6	9.6
• Three or more	6.6	2.2	4.7
Average number of sexual contacts, past 30 days[b,c]	1.0	0.6	0.8
Sexual contacts in the past 30 days, with a regular partner or with other partners			
• Regular partner	47.1	58.9	51.3
• Other partners	52.9	41.1	48.8

[a] Significant difference: $\alpha = 5\%$

[b] Highly significant difference: $\alpha = 1\%$

[c] The average was based on the gross values of the variables

month. More users (53 percent) than nonusers (41 percent) said they had sex in the past month with someone other than their usual partner.

However, not having a stable partner does not seem to be a key reason for frequenting PSPs. Of those who do visit public places, 22 percent said they had not had a stable partner in the past twelve months, as compared to 29 percent of those who do not visit PSPs. Also, 45 percent of those who visit PSPs, and 51 percent of those who do not, had a stable partner over the same period.

Those who visit public sex places tend to be better at sexual communication than those who do not (see Table 5.7). The differences between users and nonusers became readily apparent when it came to oral sex. Those who visit public sex places find it easier to convey to their partners whether they want their nipples sucked or not, whether it is all right to ejaculate in the mouth, and whether to use a condom during oral sex. This suggests that visiting parks and other public spaces increases the ability to communicate about oral sex; an alternative explanation would be that men who like to engage in public sex are also those who are more open about their enjoyment of oral sex and can communicate their desires more effectively.

TABLE 5.7. Ability to Communicate About Sexual Matters, As Related to Use or Nonuse of Public Sex Places

	Very easy to easy		**Normal**		**Difficult to very difficult**	
	User	Non-User	User	Non-User	User	Non-User
Asking someone to have a sexual encounter	32.9	24.8	18.9	18.2	48.2	56.9
Being asked to have a sexual encounter	42.4	32.8	24.4	18.2	22.5	48.9
Asking someone to engage in passive oral sex without a condom**	35.4	20.4	14.0	5.0	50.6	71.5
Asking someone to engage in passive oral sex with a condom	40.9	35.8	12.2	13.1	47.0	51.1
Asking someone to engage in active oral sex without a condom**	49.4	31.4	7.9	10.9	42.7	57.7

Asking someone to engage in active oral sex with a condom	35.4	36.5	11.6	14.6	53.0	48.9
Asking someone to engage in passive oral sex and ejaculate in the mouth	6.1	5.8	2.4	15.2	91.5	92.7
Asking someone to engage in passive oral sex and not ejaculate in the mouth**	42.4	16.8	9.5	15.3	48.2	67.9
Asking someone to engage in active oral sex and ejaculate in the mouth**	23.2	13.9	7.9	5.1	38.9	81.0
Asking someone to engage in active oral sex and not ejaculate in the mouth**	43.9	25.5	10.4	13.9	45.7	60.6
Expressing the desire to penetrate the other person while using a condom	59.8	53.3	7.9	7.3	32.3	39.4
Expressing the desire to penetrate the other person without using a condom	13.4	8.1	1.8	1.5	84.8	90.4
Expressing the desire to be penetrated with a condom	37.8	30.1	7.3	8.1	54.9	61.8
Expressing the desire to be penetrated without a condom	7.9	5.2	1.8	3.0	93.3	91.9
Expressing the desire to ejaculate within the other person**	29.9	16.9	5.5	5.9	64.6	77.2
Expressing the desire to be penetrated and for the other person to ejaculate within you	13.6	6.7	4.3	5.2	82.1	88.1
Expressing the desire to be penetrated without any internal ejaculation	19.5	14.5	9.4	9.9	71.1	75.6
Performing oral sex on the partner, without a condom, after the partner has performed a penetration	1.2	3.7	2.4	1.5	96.3	94.9
Performing oral sex on the partner, with a condom, after the partner has performed a penetration	7.7	8.1	6.1	1.5	86.6	90.4
Licking the anus of a partner who has been penetrated	7.9	5.9	4.3	—	87.8	94.1
Licking the partner's nipples**	82.9	66.2	8.2	12.5	8.5	21.6
Being kissed on the mouth*	84.1	67.2	7.3	15.3	8.5	17.5

TABLE 5.7 (*continued*)

	Very easy to easy		**Normal**		**Difficult to very difficult**	
	User	Non-User	User	Non-User	User	Non-User
Not being kissed on the mouth	36.6	37.5	21.1	25.7	42.2	36.8
Asking the partner whether he has a sexually transmitted disease	46.3	58.8	11.6	5.1	42.1	36.0
Asking the partner whether he suffers from AIDS/HIV	45.1	56.2	9.1	3.6	45.7	40.1
Telling the partner that a part of his body smells	51.8	66.4	14.0	2.9	34.1	30.7
Asking the partner to wash before a sexual encounter	67.1	77.4	14.6	9.5	18.3	13.1
Telling the partner that he smells	58.8	69.3	11.6	5.1	29.9	25.5
Asking the partner to wash his penis if it smells	71.0	68.6	9.9	7.3	19.1	24.1
Telling the partner that one wishes to use objects in the sexual encounter	26.8	21.2	8.5	7.3	64.6	71.5
Telling the partner that one does not wish to use objects in the sexual encounter	58.5	65.0	11.6	8.8	29.9	26.3

* Significant difference: $\alpha = 5\%$
** Highly significant difference: $\alpha = 1\%$

When asked for the reasons to visit public sex places, significant differences were observed between those who visit them and those who do not (see Table 5.8). Those who use PSPs find them significantly more erotic because of the degree of danger involved (30.6 percent of those who engage in public sex thought so, as opposed to 23.4 percent among those who do not). Regular users are also more likely to say they feel uncontrollable urges to engage in sex: 41.5 percent, compared to 19.3 percent. They are also more likely to say they enjoy having sex with strangers (29.8 percent versus 12.4 percent), as well as group sex (15.3 percent versus 6.3 percent). Finally, only a small minority claimed that they visit public sex places because they feel unattractive.

TABLE 5.8. Distribution of Variables Related to Desire to Have Sexual Relations, As Related to Use or Nonuse of Public Sex Places

	Visits PSPs	Does not visit PSPs	Total
(N)	(164)	(137)	(301)
TOTAL	100	100	100
The sense of danger makes the sexual encounter more exciting**			
• Agree	30.6	23.4	30.2
• Disagree	58.5	66.4	62.1
• Not sure	5.5	10.5	7.6
Feel uncontrollable desires to engage in sexual encounters**			
• Always or nearly always	41.5	19.3	31.2
• Sometimes	41.7	48.9	45.0
• Never or almost never	17.2	31.9	23.9
Give in to these desires			
• Always or nearly always	47.2	30.2	38.2
• Sometimes	42.9	49.1	45.6
• Never or almost never	13.8	20.7	16.1
Ways of satisfying such desires (N)	(113)	(151)	(264)
Masturbates			
• Yes (spontaneous response)	70.2	71.7	70.8
• Yes (after prompting)	20.5	17.7	19.3
• No	9.3	10.6	9.8
Engages in sex with his stable partner			
• Yes (spontaneous response)	23.2	24.8	23.9
• Yes (after prompting)	25.2	29.2	26.9
• No	51.7	46.2	49.2
Engages in sex with an acquaintance**			
• Yes (spontaneous response)	15.9	7.1	12.1
• Yes (after prompting)	34.4	29.2	29.9
• No	49.7	46.2	58.8
Engages in sex with a stranger**			
• Yes (spontaneous response)	6.0	2.7	4.5
• Yes (after prompting)	23.8	9.7	17.8
• No	70.2	87.9	77.7

TABLE 5.8 (*continued*)

		Visits PSPs	Does not visit PSPs	Total
Ways of satisfying such desires	**(N)**	**(113)**	**(151)**	**(264)**
Engages in group sex*				
• Yes (spontaneous response)		0.7	0.9	0.8
• Yes (after prompting)		14.6	5.4	10.6
• No		84.8	93.8	88.6
Considers himself to be attractive				
• Very attractive or attractive		31.7	29.9	30.9
• Normal		51.8	48.9	50.5
• Unattractive or very unattractive		16.4	21.2	18.6

* Significant difference: $\alpha = 5\%$
** Highly significant difference: $\alpha = 1\%$

Having sex with strangers is an additional attraction for the clients of public places. That much is clear. However, what is meant by the "sense of danger"? Gay life in Costa Rica implies a number of hazards in any case, so it is hardly surprising that people who had their sexual initiation in these places might have acquired a taste for the risks involved in such a liaison. Kenneth explains:

> I'm worried that this is becoming a need. It's like an addiction that I can't stop. When I don't come here for a few days, I feel like I'm drowning. I come here without telling my lover, but some of my friends—people he doesn't know—have told me that they've seen him hanging around here, cruising. You may think I'm a bit of a masochist, and maybe you're right. Maybe I'm looking to get killed. Did you ever see a movie called *Looking for Mr. Goodbar,* with Diane Keaton? I loved that movie and I really identified with the main character. If you ever run across my name in the paper, in the obituary section, you'll know how I died.

Juan, a chauffeur, had this to say:

> I do this often. It's like an addiction, 'cause I have a lover and we get along real well. The problem is, we only see each other

> on weekends, because he lives out of town. In the middle of the week, this is where I come to get my kicks. But I tell you, it's very dangerous. You can't be completely sure of who's getting into the car with you. There's so many criminals around. . . . I get a kick out of the sense of danger.

Heriberto agrees:

> Behind the park there's a dark alleyway where I've seen many things happen. A lot of guys arrive in their cars, park them, and go in there. It's a very dangerous place. It's very exciting to be there. I find fear exciting, the idea that the police might show up, or a private guard. . . . I like that sense of fear.

Part of the thrill comes from the feeling of the forbidden and from being hurried. "There's no need for long conversations and fancy courtships," says Mario.

Some gay men who are regular clients of the movie theaters admit that they find the fear of exposure to be an exciting turn-on. One of them explains:

> Once I was talking to a friend who likes to go there (to a particular theater) and he told me that for him it is like going on a safari, a kind of escape. He told me some experiences he'd had in the theater that made my hair stand on end. I could hardly believe what he told me, but it might just be true. . . .

Table 5.9 confirms these responses. When asked for the main reason why they frequented public sex places, 63.4 percent mentioned having sex without any strings attached, 54.9 percent spoke of the speed with which one could "score," 53.7 percent mentioned the pleasure of meeting new people, 48.2 percent said they enjoyed doing something "forbidden," 46.3 percent said they enjoyed watching other people having sex, 45.1 percent claimed they felt excited by the danger of being discovered, and 40.2 percent mentioned quick sex.

One attraction of the PSPs is to meet men who do not go to gay bars. Only a small minority of the gay community in Costa Rica go

TABLE 5.9. Reasons for Visiting Public Sex Places

(N)	**(164)**
Reason for visiting public sex places	
• Engaging in sex with no strings attached	63.4
• Having the chance to score quickly with someone	54.9
• Feeling the constant need to meet new people	53.7
• Doing something considered taboo	48.2
• Enjoying the sight of other people engaging in sex	46.3
• Enjoying the danger of being found out	45.1
• Enjoying a "quickie"	40.2
• Feeling lonely	38.4
• Enjoying the feeling of putting oneself at risk because of the choice of venue	36.6
• Having sex with strangers	36.0
• Drinking alcohol	34.8
• Being able to have sex without engaging in small talk	30.5
• Having most sexual contacts in public places	27.0
• Finding it difficult to score in bars or discos	25.0
• Feeling unattractive	23.8
• Having sex with different people each time	22.1
• Being able to pay to have sex with someone	21.3
• Not wanting to be identified as a homosexual	20.9
• Having sex with more than one person at a time	15.9
• Wanting others to watch while one is engaging in sex	11.6
• Having sex with aggressive individuals	9.1
• Making money	5.5
• Taking drugs	3.7
Motivation index for visiting public sex places*	
• Average	4.0
• Mode	0.0
• Medium	3.0
Frequency of visits to public sex places	
• More than twice a week	25.0
• Once a week	11.6
• Once a month	22.6
• A few times a year	40.9

ACTIVITIES CARRIED OUT IN PSPs

Watching	
• Yes (spontaneous response)	45.7
• Yes (after prompting)	32.3
• No	22.0
Making friends	
• Yes (spontaneous response)	25.6
• Yes (after prompting)	37.2
• No	37.2
Masturbating someone	
• Yes (spontaneous response)	17.1
• Yes (after prompting)	32.9
• No	50.0
Having someone masturbate you	
• Yes (spontaneous response)	16.5
• Yes (after prompting)	37.8
• No	45.7
Performing oral sex on someone	
• Yes (spontaneous response)	7.3
• Yes (after prompting)	24.4
• No	68.3
Receiving oral sex from someone	
• Yes (spontaneous response)	13.4
• Yes (after prompting)	40.2
• No	46.3
Penetrating someone	
• Yes (spontaneous response)	5.5
• Yes (after prompting)	18.9
• No	75.6
Being penetrated by someone	
• Yes (spontaneous response)	1.8
• Yes (after prompting)	11.0
• No	87.2
Going off to someone's house	
• Yes (spontaneous response)	1.2
• Yes (after prompting)	28.7
• No	70.1
Taking someone to one's own house	
• Yes (spontaneous response)	0.6
• Yes (after prompting)	21.5
• No	77.9

* The index was estimated by adding all affirmative responses to the question. Minimum value is 0 (zero); maximum value is 24.

to bars that cater specifically to this clientele. Public sex places, therefore, offer "new faces," including men who have not yet come out of the closet. Many gays are excited by this idea. This is evident in the number of bisexual men who use these places as their only source of nonheterosexual satisfaction:

> I don't know why I do it. It's an urge that's stronger than me. I don't understand what's happening. I have a great sex life at home. I make love very often. But about once every six weeks, my desires build up and then I need to make love with a man. . . .

Another attraction is the chance to make friends. As shown in Table 5.9, almost 63 percent of respondents say that this is the main reason they visit public places. With respect to saunas, the openly gay males who visit them do so to make friends and have sex without the complex mating rituals that often take place in bars. The sense of danger that often comes with the experience of visiting other public sex places does not apply in this instance, since saunas are not raided by the police:

> I don't really know why I come to places like this. Maybe it's loneliness, and it gets to be too much of a burden sometimes. . . . It upsets me that gay people should be submerged in a world of fiction. . . . When you go to bars, they're always talking about traveling, about cars, things like that, even when they don't have a cent. You're judged by the designer brand on your pants or your shirt. Here, we all know what we came for; everything is much simpler.

Other significant reasons include watching others having sex (78 percent), being masturbated (54.3 percent), receiving oral sex (53.6 percent), and masturbating someone (50 percent) (see Table 5.9). It is worth noting that more than 35 percent of those who visit PSPS say they do so once a week at least.

When we asked both groups to assess different places according to their degree of erotic appeal (see Table 5.10), we found that the preferred locations for both groups were public toilets, parks, alleyways, movie theaters, saunas, and vehicles, in that order. The places

TABLE 5.10. Average of the Ten Most Erotic Places for Sex, As Related to Use or Nonuse of Public Sex Places

Place	Visits PSPs	Does not visit PSPs	Total
Homes*	3.93	2.40	3.23
Apartments**	3.58	2.91	3.28
Countryside	4.72	4.23	4.50
Motels	4.73	4.30	4.53
Vehicles	4.60	4.89	4.73
Saunas*	5.07	6.11	5.54
Movie theaters**	5.33	6.93	6.60
Alleyways*	5.77	7.44	7.07
Parks	6.93	7.32	7.11
Public toilets	7.89	8.44	8.37

* Highly significant difference: $\alpha = 1\%$
** Significant difference: $\alpha = 5\%$

Note: Respondents were asked to grade each place on a scale of one to ten, with one meaning "most erotic" and ten "least erotic."

considered least erotic were people's homes, apartments, the countryside, motels, and vehicles, in that order. However, those who do not visit PSPs consider them more erotic than those who do, while the latter find private places more erotic. In other words, each group imagines that the grass is always greener on the other side of the fence. The nonparticipants tend to fantasize that public spaces are more erotic. These findings contradict Carrier's assertions about public sex in Guadalajara, Mexico. According to this anthropologist, the gays in that city have sex in public places because they do not have private apartments, which they consider their favorite place for having sex.[1]

With respect to the dangers of HIV infection, only 25 percent of those who had visited public sex places had engaged in anal penetration during their last visit, even though 45 percent had consumed alcohol before the visit. Of those who did engage in anal penetration, 83.3 percent had used a condom. Moreover, 75 percent said they never penetrate anyone, much less allow anyone to penetrate them (see Table 5.11). Although the data refer exclusively to the last visit to a public place, this suggests that penetration is not the most

TABLE 5.11. Distribution of the Variables Associated with the Use or Nonuse of Condoms and the Consumption of Alcohol and Drugs in Public Sex Places

Variables		Total
	(N)	(164)
Percentage who practiced penetration the last time that they visited an anonymous public sex place		25.6
	(N)	(42)
Percentage who used a condom the last time they visited an anonymous public sex place		83.3
Person who used the condom		
The interviewee		45.7
The sexual partner		28.6
Both		25.7
Percentage of people who consumed alcohol the last time they visited an anonymous public sex place		45.7
Percentage of people who took drugs the last time they visited an anonymous public sex place		6.1

popular practice and that, when it takes place, the majority use condoms. The ethnographic information collected so far seems to confirm this: public sex places do not stand out as focal points of unsafe sex.

In general, the favorite sexual activities are mutual masturbation and oral sex. In places such as parks, public toilets, or alleyways, the danger of being discovered or exposed is so great that this discourages anal sex.

In the case of saunas and movie theaters, the fact that such establishments are exclusively homosexual, or benefit from the indifference of their owners, allows them to be the setting for longer-lasting sexual activities, such as orgies or anal sex. In spite of this, some establishments, more than others, are the scene of more dangerous practices, as far as the risk of HIV infection is concerned. However, the fact that saunas have private cubicles makes it impossible to estimate how common such practices might be.

One factor to take into account when assessing the degree of risk found in each place has to do with the type of clientele. When clients are professionals with high levels of education, this may tend to discourage them from risky sexual practices. Another factor may be the attitude of the management toward unsafe sex. Some establishments display notices about safe sex and are more willing to distribute information or leaflets. Where this occurs, unsafe sex is discouraged.

In parks, the most common practice is mutual masturbation. But oral sex is common too, says Guillermo, a client. Even anal penetration is sometimes practiced:

> Yesterday I saw something that left me stunned. On a bench close to where I was, there was a guy sitting with his penis hanging out. Suddenly, another guy came up to me and said, "Look how great that thing is," and would I like to sit on him? I thought he was kidding, because he's a lawyer and looks very respectable. Besides, I had seen him handing out information [on safe sex] in bars. I pretended to continue the joke and said to him, "Why don't you go sit on that guy?" Next thing I knew, he went right ahead and sat on the guy. What amazed me was that they didn't say a word. The guy just pulled down his pants and the other guy just started shoving it in without any protection, without a condom. They carried on until the other guy came.

A similar story is told by Ernesto, another regular visitor to the park:

> In the darkest part [of the park], I once got to see very late at night, maybe around three in the morning, how they fucked a guy. Just imagine, the guy . . . well, I was turning the corner when I saw the edge of a small bush that someone was holding onto and he was kind of shoving into the bush. I looked more closely and I saw that the guy was being fucked by some other guy. It was something anyone could have seen if they were paying attention.

People who get into other men's cars may have oral sex or masturbate each other inside the vehicle, but most often they drive to a far-removed spot, have sex, and then return to the same park, where the passenger gets out.

In public toilets, mutual masturbation and oral sex are the most common practices. However, on one occasion our researchers saw a man in his forties taking a condom out of its package and putting it on his penis. He was about to penetrate another man whose pants were down. When they were just getting started, a heterosexual walked into the toilet. The couple quickly pretended they were doing something else and walked out of the dark toilet. Outside, they spoke and went off together.

Gerardo says that unsafe sex is practiced occasionally:

> . . . A friend told me recently that he went past a bus stop, around seven in the evening, and there was this young guy, maybe nineteen years old, with a big dick, and there was this other guy who asked him to fuck him. He pulled down his trousers and he pulled his underwear to one side over his butt, and the guy fucked him. My friend says they did it without a condom, without anything . . .

However, these are exceptional cases, says Heriberto:

> They didn't use a condom in the anal penetrations that I've seen, but you could say that most times people just play around with the other's genitals, get turned on, and then ejaculate. Every so often there are daring people who have oral sex, but that is not usual. Generally, what happens is that people masturbate each other, ejaculate, and that's the end of the coupling, if you can call it a coupling, since it's not a full coupling. . . .

Mutual masturbation is very common in movie theaters. However, the ethnographer witnessed a few rare instances of anal sex performed without a condom. One incident deserves mention: once, on the second floor of a theater, a young man between eighteen and twenty years old was penetrated successively by six men who stood in line. None used a condom. This took place in an area near the staircase. About ten other men were watching, masturbating themselves or each other.

In saunas, mutual masturbation and oral sex are also the most common practices, though the ethnographer also reports cases of penetration without the use of a condom. Others, however, insist that condoms are more widely used than in movie theaters and other public places. "I don't like using it. But it's the same as drivers who don't like wearing a safety belt. It can save your life," says Gilberto, a client.

The theoretical model we are discussing here ("of the body and its pleasures") is based on the satisfaction of the senses and of desires. The gays who hang around in bars and visit public places do so as an additional stimulus to their sex life. They are young men, aware of their homosexuality, well educated, attractive, and capable of good sexual communication. For the most part, they engage in safe sex and take precautions, mindful of the risks they face in such places. However, as we shall see in the next chapter, there are other possible reasons for visiting public sex places: these may serve as a stage for the reenactment of sexual traumas—some of them unconscious—as a way of coping with some of the participants' inner conflicts.

Chapter 6

Violence and Public Sex

An additional element suggests that the model of the body and its pleasures includes motivations other than the satisfaction of the senses. It is violence.

Table 6.1 shows that there is a significant difference between those who regularly visit public sex places and those who do not, with respect to exposure to sexual violence. In other words, some of those who visit PSPs have been exposed to more violence than those who do not. Important differences are evident between users and nonusers in terms of previous experience: 20.1 percent of users said they had been beaten, compared with 8 percent of nonusers; 19.5 percent of users suffered insults, compared with only 7.3 percent of nonusers; 18.3 percent of users said they were forced to have sex, compared with 9.5 percent of nonusers. In the case of insulting someone else—rather than being insulted—14 percent of PSP users admitted to it, compared with 6.6 percent of nonusers. Moreover, 13.4 percent of users had engaged in violent sex games with their partners, compared with 2.9 percent of nonusers. In all these cases, some PSP users had been exposed to more violence than nonusers.

From this data, we can draw two possible conclusions: that some of those who visit public sex places have experienced more sexual violence, or that visiting these places tends to increase sexual violence. It is more likely that the first hypothesis is correct.

Table 6.2 confirms our hypothesis that some of those who frequent public sex places were more frequently punished and sexually abused as children or teenagers than those who do not. Some PSP users have been subjected to significantly higher levels of severe emotional abuse before reaching the age of twelve: 42.1 percent of users compared

TABLE 6.1. Distribution of Variables Related to Violent Practices in Sexual Relations, As Related to Use or Nonuse of PSPs

Variables	Visits PSPs	Does not visit PSPs	Total
(N)	(164)	(137)	(301)
Has been beaten[a]	20.1	8.0	14.6
Has beaten someone[b]	11.6	4.4	8.3
Has been immobilized	11.0	7.3	9.3
Has immobilized someone	12.8	7.3	10.3
Has been insulted[a]	19.5	7.3	14.0
Has insulted someone[b]	14.0	6.6	10.6
Has been physically forced to have sex[b]	18.3	9.5	14.3
Has physically forced someone to have sex	4.9	2.2	3.7
Has practiced violent games[a]	13.4	2.9	8.6
Index of violence in sexual relations[a,c]			
Average	1.3	0.6	0.9
Mode	0.0	0.0	0.0
Median	1.0	0.0	0.0

[a] Highly significant difference (α = 1%)
[b] Significant difference (α = 5%)
[c] The index was calculated by summing up all affirmative answers to the question. The minimum value is 0 (zero); the highest is 9.

with 27 percent of nonusers. Between the ages of twelve and eighteen, 42.7 percent of users had experienced abuse as opposed to 27 percent of nonusers. Current emotional abuse by partners was also more prevalent among visitors to public sex places (3.7 percent) than among nonusers (3.6 percent). Similar significant differences were found with respect to physical abuse: 22 percent of users experienced it before the age of twelve, compared with 5.8 percent of nonusers; 17.1 percent of users reported physical abuse between the ages of twelve and eighteen, as opposed to 5.1 percent of nonusers. Finally, some visitors to public sex places have more frequently been victims of sexual violence before the age of twelve (20.1 percent) than nonvisitors (8.8 percent), and also between the ages of twelve and eighteen (15.9 percent compared with 6.6 percent).

TABLE 6.2. Distribution of Variables Related to Emotional, Physical, and Sexual Abuse, As Related to Use or Nonuse of PSPs

Variables		Visits PSPs	Does not visit PSPs	Total
	(N)	(164)	(137)	(301)
	Total	100	100	100
Severe emotional abuse				
• Before the age of 12*		42.1	27.0	35.2
• Between 12 and 18*		42.7	27.0	35.5
• Currently, by partner		3.7	3.6	3.7
• Currently, by others*		23.8	7.3	16.3
Severe physical abuse				
• Before the age of 12*		22.0	5.8	14.6
• Between 12 and 18*		17.1	5.1	11.6
• Currently, by partner		1.2	2.2	1.7
• Currently, by others*		6.7	0.7	4.0
Forced participation in sexual acts				
• Before the age of 12*		20.1	8.8	15.0
• Between 12 and 18*		15.9	6.6	11.6
• Currently, by partner		1.8	0.7	1.3
• Currently, by others		3.7	2.9	3.3

* Highly significant difference (α = 1%)

Some of the men who visit public sex places have suffered greater violence and abuse in their sexual relationships. Apparently, they have continued certain behavioral patterns that they learned as children and adolescents. This pattern of abuse also appears to influence their decision to visit public sex places. To understand this correlation, we brought together a group of gay men who visit public sex places and who also experienced sexual abuse and physical violence when they were children. We left out those who had suffered psychological abuse only, since it is hard to find gay men in Costa Rica who have not been exposed to this form of violence.

The forty young men who were invited to participate in a total of four workshops for gay victims of abuse between September and November 1998 were asked, among other things, to complete three specific tasks. First, they were asked to write an account of the sexual or physical abuse they had suffered as children or adolescents. The accounts of the twenty-three men who had admitted to visiting public sex places were separated from the rest. Four weeks later, the same twenty-three men were asked to describe their most erotic experiences in public places. The reason for the delay was to ensure that the participants would not make a conscious connection between the two assignments. Once these tasks were completed, however, participants were asked to read both accounts, analyze them, and write in their own words the connections they saw between the two.

The accounts included below suggest some reasons why people are attracted to public sex. However, our intention is not to suggest that there is anything pathological about public sex, nor to create the impression that these interpretations can necessarily be generalized.

Instead of viewing public sex as the result of a childhood trauma, one could look at it rather as a kind of psychodrama that allows some men to reenact some of their traumas in order to gain a greater measure of control or understanding of themselves. Perhaps public sex helps many of these young men resolve the effects of the violence suffered.

On the other hand, a clear need exists for further research on populations of men who have not been abused, yet visit public sex places. It would also be desirable to study a larger sample of abused men in order to evaluate how representative the following accounts really are.

THOU SHALT NOT COMMUNICATE (JUAN'S STORY)

The Abuse

My relationship with the gardener began when I was six years old. I remember this because I hadn't started going to school yet. He was a muscular man, a peasant, very masculine. I don't have many memories, but I do retain certain images of what we used to do. For instance, one afternoon he asked me to visit him in the garden shed where he stored his tools. In addition to the gardening tools, there was a bed in the shed. He asked me to hide with him under the bed to play for a while. The game consisted of him touching my genitals and me touching his. I remember how frightened I was when I touched his penis, and it was so enormous compared to mine. I couldn't understand how there could be so much of a difference and asked him, "How come it's so big?" He replied, "It's bigger because my dad used to stick it up my behind, and that's how it got to be so big. If you want yours to grow, I will have to stick it up you." The truth is, he didn't stick it in all the way, he would just push it around the entrance of the sphincter and make me move. I don't remember anything else. However, I felt pleasure—there was a lot in what we did. But there were also threats. The guy warned me I should never tell anyone; I should never speak. If I did, he would do the same to my mother and my sister. I could never say anything about what was going on. The relationship lasted for years. Although I tried to ask for help a few times, I was afraid that I would get punished, or that the gardener would leave me. There was affection between us, and also pleasure. But, why did we have to hide to do it? I always got the message that I couldn't talk [about it] and that what we did was improper.

The Most Erotic Experience

A year ago, I went to Pinochet Park at 9 p.m. I was walking around window-shopping, when a man in his thirties approached me. He was masculine, a rural type of guy, and he began to stare at me. He asked me what my name was and asked me if I would rather not go to a safer place, such as Parque Monumental. While we were walking toward the park he hardly said a word. However, he was touching his genitals and staring at me. He wanted to show me that he had a large penis. I can't deny I got all horny. I've always liked big penises. When we arrived, he started playing with my genitals and took me to the darkest part of the park. There he pulled down my pants and started playing with my ass. He acted as if he was going to push it up me but he didn't actually penetrate me yet. I must admit that I love feeling a penis on my backside, but I don't enjoy penetration. My great pleasure is the foreplay. When he actually started penetrating me, the pain was very great. I wasn't enjoying it. On a few previous occasions, I'd kept quiet about the pain.

But this time, when the guy was trying to get inside me, two other men approached. One of them, when he saw the pain on my face, said to him, "Don't be such an animal! Can't you see it's hurting him? Take it out and come outside him!" The guy obeyed and I enjoyed myself a lot. From that time on, I learned how to say exactly what I wanted to do.

Juan's Analysis

Now that I read my sexual experience when I was a kid and look at my erotic tastes, I find a few things in common:

- I like having sex in places that are hidden away and dark but connected to greenery: the garden shed or a public park.
- I like big penises: the gardener is the model.
- I like to have my ass fondled but not to be penetrated: similar to what I used to do as a child.
- I have problems asking clearly for what I want. However, the experiences in the park are helping me to learn how to speak out. The abuse I suffered was that I was told to shut up. The park has helped me to overcome this.

INVADED BODIES (ALBERTO'S STORY)

The Abuse

When I was ten years old, my uncle fucked me. It happened one night on a weekend, when my father and mother had gone to the movies. The only people in my house were my sister, who was eight years old, and myself. My uncle was around twenty-five years old and did not live in San José. He was still living with his parents in San Isidro de Heredia. He would sometimes visit us at our house in the capital and stay overnight in the guest room. I liked my uncle a lot because he was younger than my dad and he would take us to the movies and to eat ice cream. He had a girlfriend, Anita, who used to visit him at home. That weekend, they were alone in the guest room and the door was locked. I could hear a kind of sighing in the room but did not understand what was going on. Now I think he was trying to fuck her in there. I only managed to hear that he said to her, "Let me do it, honey, let me do it!" and she said, "No, I can't. Don't do it. It hurts." All of a sudden, Anita left the room and ran out of the house. My uncle followed her and they said something to each other outside, but I couldn't make out what it was. It was dark by now and I was in my bed. A few minutes later, my uncle came into the room and asked me if I wanted to sleep with him in his bed. I said yes and did not think there was anything wrong, because I'd done it before. When I got into his bed, he started playing with me and I realized that he was naked. I asked him not to touch me anymore but he didn't pay any attention. Soon he put some gel on his dick and he grabbed me and covered my mouth. I felt a horrible pain and tried to get away but couldn't. I don't remember anything more. I know he did it a few times and he always threatened to kill me if I told my parents. I never did. I was never able to sleep well again because I suffered from nightmares. I believed the devil was going to punish me for what I did.

The Most Erotic Experience

It happened two years ago at the La Llanura Park. I arrived and parked my car near the soccer field. I noticed a group of men in a circle. When I got closer, I could see a fairly attractive guy fucking this sixteen-year-old kid. I get excited when I see a kid getting it from behind. It's a kind of sadism I have. Since the kid was complaining that it hurt, it made me feel even hornier. I got close to the couple and started kissing the guy who was penetrating the kid. I felt very attracted to him. After a while two of the guys who were watching walked up to me and asked me why I didn't give my ass to the guy I was kissing. Without giving me a chance to say anything, they tore off my clothes between them. I felt ashamed but I also felt great pleasure when they pulled down my pants and made me bend over. The guy took his penis out of the kid and started fucking me. I felt a lot of pain but also great satisfaction because I felt humiliated, used, treated like a whore. However, when one of the two guys tried to do the same to me I told him no, that I didn't want to, and I didn't let him. I didn't like the guy and I wasn't going to let him fuck me.

Alberto's Analysis

What is similar about these two stories? Well, the first thing is that I like to be treated like a whore. My uncle came after me because his girlfriends wouldn't give him what he wanted. And I didn't have the power to say no to him. Besides, why deny it? I liked him. That's why, when I get treated like a vulgar whore, I get really turned on. I realize that I like being the substitute. Just like I gave my uncle the piece of ass that Anita refused to let him have, I also like it when the guy who's fucking someone else moves on to me and treats me like a substitute. Deep down, I guess I see my role as "the other." It made me feel superior to Anita and to his other girlfriends.

Finally, I see that I like being told what to do, for people to take my body without asking permission. When the guys took off my clothes, it was a real turn-on. They didn't give a damn what I wanted, they just wanted to watch a live porn movie. I've always responded according to what other people wanted from me. I guess I learned that from my uncle: my body can be invaded without my consent.

Even though I enjoy it, I feel I can stop when things aren't going the way I want them to. I realize I felt a great satisfaction when I told the guy that I didn't want him to fuck me. I may be a cheap whore, but I get to choose my clients!

THE EROTICISM OF DANGER (PEPE'S STORY)

The Abuse

I don't know if I should call my story "abuse." What I do know is that when we were kids my cousins and I had sexual relations. Of the five cousins who took part, some were fifteen, sixteen, seventeen years old. The other two of us were eight and nine years old. The older ones took advantage of us and made us suck and masturbate them. They would generally give us liquor to numb us. We never tried penetration. However, several times our uncles discovered us and gave us all a beating. One time, my eight-year-old cousin and I were sucking my seventeen-year-old cousin. We were in the bathroom; he would take us there on the pretext that he had to give us a shower because we were very dirty. Once we were inside, he would take out his cock and ask us to suck it. If we refused, he would whack us. If we bit him, he would do the same. Edwin—that was his name—was the one who forced us to do this to the other older cousins. Every time he said to us that Ernesto or Pedro were going to give us a shower, we knew what he had in mind. Well, one day we were with him and Uncle Carlos, his father, came into the bathroom and found us. He gave the two of us a real beating and I was terrified that he would kill us.

The Most Erotic Experience

I have fulfilled my erotic dreams in a public toilet. Toilets really get my hormones going. I always go there drunk. I need liquor to give me the strength to do what I'm going to do there. One day I went in and there were three guys pretending to pee. I started looking at their penises and one of them, without saying anything, grabbed my head and pulled it toward his dick. I sucked him off until he came. Then the other one gave me his and I started doing the same. At that moment, another guy came into the toilet. All of us had to pretend that we were peeing, but the guy must have suspected something because he left immediately. I guessed that he wasn't a homosexual and that he might possibly report our activities to the police. I felt very frightened, because the police might burst in at any moment. I find fear very erotic. When I do things that are improper, I find them more of a turn-on. That's why I like public toilets, because there's always an element of danger. Well, that one time, the guy came and nothing happened. However, as soon as we'd finished, a cop came along to see what was going on. Since he didn't see anything suspicious, he left, and I ended up performing oral sex on the third guy. The more I realized that we had been under surveillance but we had not been caught, the more I enjoyed what I was doing.

Pepe's Analysis

Hey, I've just understood where my cock sucking comes from! Also, the reason why I always drink before I visit public toilets, and that this business of drinking must have started early. It's pretty clear that I learned to suck dick when I was little, and that I did it under the surveillance of my uncles, who must have been at least partially aware of what was going on. I also realize why public toilets really turn me on. When I was a kid, I would have sex in the bathroom and now I go to public toilets. I like to make love in places where I need to be on guard. Even when I do it in the bedroom, I'm aware of the door and the phone, as if someone might come in or call.

However, my biggest insight is that visiting dangerous places is my greatest passion. I feel that my body needs a great deal of adrenaline to enjoy sex. When I have the chance of being in a public toilet with a man, there's always uncertainty about who might come in and what they might do to us. That's just how I felt when I was in the bathroom with my cousins. But on those occasions I was really afraid of punishment. I thought they would kill me if they found out. Visiting public toilets now allows me to remember and relive that fear. However, I feel a great sense of satisfaction when I have sex in a toilet and no one catches me at it. It's sort of like telling myself, "Everything's fine; keep on sucking, 'cause you're too smart for something bad to happen to you."

NONVERBAL SEX (EMILIO'S STORY)

The Abuse

The story of my abuse happened because of my own father. I can't remember when it began, because my memory isn't too good. I suffer from mental blackouts about everything that went on during my childhood. I can only remember three occasions, when I was twelve years old, that my dad took me with him on a beach holiday. The two of us were alone in a room in some cheap hotel. You could hear everything that went on in the next room. Now I think that's the reason he took me there. My dad was still a young man (he has since died); he was about thirty-two at that time. Well, we arrived in the morning and went swimming. I had a really good time at the beach, and then we went back to the room to change. I swear I had no idea of what was going to happen. A few times before, my dad had played with me and touched my genitals, but as a joke. Looking back, I recall him saying things like, "How much you've grown!" or, "How large does it get when you get a hard-on?" But I didn't pay any attention to that. Well, we got to the room, and he asked me to get undressed so we could take a shower. When we were naked, my dad showed me his penis, which was really standing up. I was afraid, but he said that was normal when he washed himself with soap. Then he grabbed mine and asked me if I had measured how long it got when it was standing up. I said no. He pretended that he was going to examine it and he got his "medical" bag and took out a tape measure. By that time I was feeling scared and could not say a word. He came over with the tape measure and started rubbing suntan lotion on my penis and asking me to get an erection. Although I was petrified and sweating from fear, it gradually got harder, and he started sucking me off. I asked him not to do it, but he said to me, "Shut your mouth! The whole hotel will find out! Can't you see, everything you say can be heard in the next room?" I was overwhelmed by fear. The fear paralyzed me, until I could not utter a single sound.

The Most Erotic Experience

It happened in a sauna. A kid of about eighteen arrived with a friend of his. I've always been turned on by innocent teenage kids. This one was quite a little man, but he had the face of an angel. I believe it was the first time he had visited a sauna, and I was sure he was doing it out of curiosity. I noticed that he went into the steam room and I did the same. I went in and I saw that he was playing with his genitals. I came close and without saying anything I knelt down and began doing fellatio on him. It turned out that the kid was a Cuban and he talked too much. While I was sucking him he kept saying, "Enjoy it good; enjoy it!" When people are having sex with me and keep on talking, I get pissed. I can't bear to hear words. So I asked him if he wanted us to go to a cubicle. When he got into one with me, I started kissing him to shut him up. The kid said he wanted me to stick it up him. I told him then, "If you want my dick, you're going to shut up. Do you want the whole sauna to know I'm fucking you?" I spoke roughly. The little Cuban shut up and nodded that he wanted me to penetrate him. I did it but in the gentlest way imaginable: I rubbed his sphincter with a little coke that I had been hiding in my towel, so he didn't feel any pain. He told me it had been the most painless and enjoyable fuck he'd ever had.

Emilio's Analysis

I realize now that the gaps in my memory might have to do with my relationship with my father. There were other things that I don't want to remember. I also realize that I like doing to kids what my father did to me. The fact that I forced the kid to shut up, and that I enjoyed it, shows me that I'm repeating my own story. For me, sex should be performed in silence, without anyone else finding out, the way my father taught me. If I have the chance to force someone to shut his mouth, I find that more exciting. It's what my father did to me: he took me to a place where I couldn't complain or say anything. I had to protect him, as much as myself. I realize that I go for sex in places that remind me of the cheap hotel where my father initiated me. Saunas with cubicles where you can hear everything are the closest thing to that hotel. Finally, I feel as if I am responsible for the welfare of the kids I fuck, doing things gently, not the way my dad did it to me, sadistically.

THE NEED TO DISCONNECT (MIGUEL'S STORY)

The Abuse

My dad was an alcoholic. He had eight kids and could never support any of them. He couldn't keep a job for very long, and the only thing he could do was jobs like mowing lawns. I can't remember the first time he hit my mother, me, and my brothers. I think it's something that had always happened. He would come home drunk and take out his rage on her. He accused her of sleeping with other men, because he was very jealous. When he started hitting, he wouldn't stop. Since I was the oldest, I had to defend my mother and stay with her. The way I managed to do this was by disconnecting myself from the situation. I didn't feel the slaps or the howls; I didn't see the blood. I would only become aware of all this the next day. It was like being on automatic pilot: I could speak, see what was going on, but I wasn't there. My mind was somewhere in the clouds.

The Most Erotic Experience

I am a big movie fan. I love to watch a porn movie and let my desire carry me away. About three months ago I went to the Limon City Cinema to watch a hot film. The guy in it had a big dick and was fucking three women at an orgy. The guy was fairly rough and he liked to mistreat. The movie was at its hottest when I had to rush to the men's room. I saw four men waiting in there. None of them was with any of the others. The four were very masculine. When I see a sight like that, I get carried away. I approached them and dropped my pants without saying a word and I started walking around with my butt exposed. I know I should have realized how dangerous it was, but I was overcome with pleasure. I saw one of them approach me and, without asking permission, he bent me over. Once I was bent over, he told me he was a cop, and that I was under arrest for public indecency. The other three also said they were cops. However, they locked the men's room and stayed inside. One of them stuck his penis out and says to me: "So you want dick, you queen? Well, here's what you're looking for." Another one said to me, "The four of us are going to fuck you, starting with the smallest and moving on to the largest, to see how much you can take." Although technically I was being raped, I won't lie and pretend I didn't enjoy it. The four of them fucked me for about an hour. When they finally let me go, I was bleeding and in a lot of pain. However, I remember this incident and fantasize about it when I masturbate.

Miguel's Analysis

Hearing both stories again, I feel that I have a problem of disconnecting myself when it comes to sex and in many other areas of my life. Watching movies makes me enter into a state of numbness in which I look for violent and dangerous situations. It's like being in another world. Once I'm in one of these situations, my body and my brain drift apart. That's probably the same thing that happened when my dad used to beat us: my mind would leave the room and not pay attention to the damage until later. I feel the same thing happens with violent sex scenes. I realize that in both cases I end up bleeding, though my body hasn't felt the pain. However, I tell myself that I'm the one who willingly gets into these messy situations.

THE WORST NIGHTMARES

All the stories in this chapter reveal symptoms that have been identified with childhood sexual abuse. In his study of men who have been abused, Mike Lew says that victims suffer from memory loss, excessive watchfulness, problems coping with boundaries, denial of abuse, addictions to sex, drugs, or drinking to help reduce the level of pain, emotional numbing, and sleep disorders.[1] Lew also believes that if a victim does not receive treatment for his trauma, he will be forced unconsciously to reenact it in order to gain some control over it.

Some of our interviewees are aware that they reenact in public places the difficult situations they experienced as children. It is likely that visiting such places has helped them to improve their sexual openness and ability to communicate. In this respect, the experience of "playing" and of meeting different men is positive. Reenacting traumatic experiences allows them to "resolve" them, or at least experience them from an adult perspective, without the vulnerability associated with childhood.

However, as we shall see in the next chapter, these places are fraught with great danger. If gay men do not realize that the model of the body and its pleasures is only one of several sexual models present in public places, they may find that their best fantasies can turn into their worst nightmares.

Chapter 7

Cacheros and Locusts (*Chapulines*)

In the movie *Fiddler on the Roof,* we are initially shown images full of color and music to convey to us the supposedly bucolic life of the Jewish communities of eastern Europe. However, the music and color soon subside, introducing the "others," the problematic Christians, many of them anti-Semitic. If it were not for them, the movie suggests, life in Russia or Poland would not have been so tragic for this persecuted minority. Nevertheless, Levinas tells us that the look of the "other" determines our knowledge of ourselves. Without the other, we are nothing.[1]

We must do the same. We must also show the "others." If it were not for them, the gays would have a fantastic time in public places, dancing and cavorting in response to the call of Eros. However, like birds of ill omen, there are vultures who circle in the sky waiting to disrupt homosexual pleasures. They share a common background, being from the poorer and least educated classes of society. The majority have not even completed second grade in primary school. Many are illiterate. A large group of them have no home and sleep in parks and vacant lots. They come from broken families, the result of a lack of sexual education that is part of the Catholic Church's demographic terrorism. Most have multiple addictions: glue, marijuana, crack, alcohol, and cigarettes. Nobody wants them and the middle classes dream of some calamity that will wipe them all out. The average life span of these poor devils is extremely short. According to Antonio Bustamante, coordinator of ILPES' AIDS-prevention program—the only one of its kind for this group—"most are dead before the age of twenty-five."

It is important to understand that their perceptions of homosexuality differ greatly from those of homosexuals themselves. Among

Latin America's lower classes, homosexuality is not seen as a psychological condition. The idea that our sexuality is somehow "hidden" in our heads, as modern psychology theorizes, is incomprehensible to them. That view is more in line with the ideas of the middle classes, for whom nonphysical attributes such as class and education are important.

For the masses, it is the tangible things and the things that they lack which are important: a home, clothing, food, and of course, control over their own bodies. In his analysis of the relationship between modern life and insanity, Louis A. Sass tells us that it was not until the sixteenth century that people began to believe that a difference exists between personality and activity.[2] Given that ancient and medieval societies were static and people could not change their occupation or their social status, the concept that one could be something other than what one did or did not do with one's body was nonexistent. There was no awareness of the idea that something in our heads could differ from what we did socially and that it was somehow independent and more "real." Thus, Sass concludes that social mobility, promoted by economic development and "modernity," was largely responsible for people beginning to consider the personality as something internal and as something changing and pliable, that could be cultivated, educated, and developed. For the lower classes of society, whether medieval or modern, who lack opportunities to change and improve their career and social position, and the opportunity to cultivate their internal selves, this notion remains problematic or incomprehensible.

Foucault believes that homosexuality is a recent creation linked to modernity.[3] The discovery of homosexuality (or its invention) was associated, from the start, with the medical desire to study it and regulate it. In other words, people began to be divided according to the object of our sexual desire (something not done previously), and some could be considered as suffering from a sexual disorder. This suggests that we were not always categorized by the objects of our desire. In fact, in Classical Greece, citizens could change sexual objects without any problem. However, what could not be done was to change practices: honorable men could not allow themselves to be penetrated. But they could penetrate women, men, and beasts. [4]

For young street kids, as for ancient Greeks, homosexuality is an inversion of gender that has nothing to do with psychological development. Homosexuals are those who exchange the masculine for the feminine. A man is heterosexual so long as he is masculine and the same holds true for women so long as they are feminine. Thus, *cacheros*[5] and locusts[6] are not perceived as homosexuals, nor is the idea of a specific "psychology" or inner world accepted.

Young people and adults from marginal communities who have few opportunities to study, make money, and be socially mobile exercise power through the only means they have at their disposal: their bodies. Gender is defined by the body, which is at the center of the battle for control. When these young people are asked how a woman should dress, they generally answer, "very feminine": short dresses, shorts, tight-fitting blouses. Men should dress in a masculine way: pants, shirts, "macho" clothes. Women should swing their bodies as they walk, but men should walk straight. Their voices should be distinctive: refined and gentle ones for women, deep and harsh ones for men. The same is true of sexual orientation. Since homosexuality is centered in the body, it is visible in people's mannerisms. Desire is not a subjective experience, but a chemical substance that, according to Alberto, a young criminal, is found in the rectum: "Faggots develop hormones in their asses which make them enjoy anal sex."

Among the lower classes, then, sexuality is not defined by the object of sexual desire. The world is not divided according to psychological attributes, but rather according to who dominates whom. All individuals who are "active" or "aggressive" are men and all those who are "passive" and who are "dominated" are women. Gender and even sexual orientation are determined by physical activity.

When these people discuss how others became homosexual they conclude that it is the result of a confusion of the active or masculine activities with passive or feminine ones. Men become homosexual because they spent too much time playing with women's things, and women become lesbians for the opposite reason. Asking a young man to clean the house or wash clothes may change his sexual orientation.

In everyone's eyes then, "faggots" or homosexuals are "women," while "dykes" or lesbians are "men" in women's bodies. Individuals who do not fit into this pattern—in other words, *cacheros* and the feminine lovers of "dykes"—do not belong to a category different from heterosexuality. In this way, the contradictions are made invisible and the world remains polarized between the strong and the weak. The machismo that is prevalent among Costa Rica's lower classes is very different from the type encountered by Mirandé in the Hispanic communities of the United States, where it is related to family values, loyalty, and religious views.[7]

The model of vulnerable masculinity applies more to communities where the traditional discourses are in crisis and men feel increasingly threatened by unemployment and their capacity to head their households. The exercise of physical force becomes the last weapon to preserve the prerogatives of gender. Men become men through violence and the subjugation of women or of other men. Males are trained from childhood to touch, abuse, mock, silence, force, subjugate, persuade, and finally rape women.

CACHEROS

When we conducted the ethnographic survey in 1989 we found two marginal subcultures in public sex places. The first group were the *cacheros* who worked in prostitution. In Latin mass culture, these men are not considered homosexual, so long as they are the penetrators in anal sex, in theory or in appearance. Given that activity and passivity determine gender among the lower classes, *cacheros* are regarded as active and therefore masculine. For them, the motivation is to earn money from sex.

Many had their own specific pickup points. But if business was slow and there were no clients, the easiest way to find them was to go to parks, toilets, alleyways, and movie theaters:

> I saw a queen pay a guy 1,000 colones to suck him. The guy was smoking a marijuana joint in a doorway with his dick hanging out. After sucking him, the queen paid him. (Victor)

Others went to public places, made their contacts and, once they were at the client's hotel or apartment, they would put their cards on the table and discuss the price to be charged for various sexual activities. Sex workers tended to prefer men who arrived in cars, since it was easier to negotiate in another place than in the pickup areas.

> I was very horny that night and went for a drive around the park. I met a very attractive young man who stared at me as I stopped at the lights. When I drove around again, he got in the car and it wasn't till we got to my apartment that he told me what he charged and explained that the price would vary according to what we did. (Luis)

Sex workers committed crimes only when clients refused to pay them the agreed sum or when they got drunk or stoned and became careless. After all, it was not in their interest to be branded as thieves. Getting clients depended on providing a good service, and a reputation as a mugger would drive them out of the market.

There was another more peculiar group, the common delinquents:

> There is a bunch of hoodlums here. I would never take any of them to my apartment. I did it once and they stole my things, but the sense of danger attracts me. (Gerardo)

> Someone told me that once, in the park, a guy took out a knife and stole his gun. I'm telling you this so you can see that in these places there are weapons and people are frightened, really scared. Then the guy showed me a large knife. I froze and stepped back. That was something that scared me. To hide my fear, I talked to him the way he talked. I got down to his level. It's a way of making yourself out to be part of the same group, the same social and cultural stratum, if you can call it that. (Eduardo)

A man named Carlos was mugged twice. Another man, José, recounts his experience:

> On February 16, 1990, I was looking for adventure in the park. It was around two in the morning. At the edge of the sidewalk I found a kid of about eighteen. He was crying. I went over to him and he said that he'd just been mugged by a couple of

> guys. They'd taken out a knife and had stolen his watch, his shirt, jewelry, money, and worst of all, they'd left him without his shoes. He was distraught and very nervous. He lived far from San José and didn't even have money for a cab. Since I had my car, I offered to take him home. I said I'd leave him a couple of blocks from his house to avoid getting involved in any problems he might have with his family.

During an observation in the park, the ethnographer, in the company of some friends, saw a known deaf gay man walking around the area for several hours. The next day, one of the friends told the ethnographer that the deaf man was in the hospital. He had been mugged at 2:00 that morning, and had been stabbed twice in his stomach and once in his neck. Another gay man was mugged the next day. They held a knife to his throat and stole all his valuables.

Another common practice by muggers in those places was to steal people's wallets while they were having oral sex. In the toilet, on January 14, 1990, at 8:00 in the evening, the ethnographer saw a man, who was giving oral sex to another, take money out of his pants. When the ethnographer tried to warn the victim that he was being robbed, a third individual approached him and put a knife against his back, warning him in a low voice: "Keep quiet." The ethnographer left without being able to do anything.

Jesús reports a similar incident:

> Once after a party, a friend of mine and I decided to take a walk around the park. We were really drunk and he decided to enter the park. I didn't want to go in. About five days later, I met him in San José and he told me that he'd been mugged that night. He was left in his underpants. He had to wait for someone to find him a taxi.

Ignacio told us:

> The first time I was robbed was about six or seven years ago. I'd just come out of a disco and went to the park. A guy came up to me, a black guy who sells lottery tickets now. I felt a certain mistrust because he used a kind of jargon that I don't use. I was a little drunk, but not too crazy. I began talking with

> the guy. He said he had an apartment near the hospital, by the railroad line, and invited me back for a drink. He tried to get information about where I worked and my name, very insistently. I gave him a false name and a false workplace. He repeatedly asked me for my phone number at work, but I didn't give it to him. Before reaching the apartment he said the place might be occupied by a gringa friend. If it was occupied, he said, a light would be on. He made a show of arriving at the apartment, and a light was on. He said we should go to an uninhabited area near the hospital. We went there and he began to suck me and I began to touch him. My wallet dropped out of my back pocket and I put it back in again. As my pants were halfway down my legs, the guy grabbed my wallet and said he would take care of it. I trusted him. But after a while I began to feel uneasy and became nervous. I had a lot of money on me that day. He didn't want to return the wallet. He turned and said, "I've just escaped from La Reforma [the jail], so I'm going to take this." In the end I persuaded him to leave me some money. He gave me 500 colones and the wallet and ran off. I felt real bad and I cried.

Carlos had a similar experience:

> Another time, when I was very drunk, completely intoxicated, I saw a guy crossing the park. He came up to me and said we should talk. I didn't like him much, but maybe because of the booze, my instinct sort of deserted me. A few days later I met him again. I didn't remember him from before. I was very drunk and we walked. He took me to the same place as before. We masturbated. He was sucking me and took out my wallet. I saw him. He was bending down and I was standing. I didn't do anything because I was so drunk that I thought if I did something this guy would kill me. I thought it was better for him to take the money and not hurt me. Very skillfully, he took the wallet out of my pants, removed the bills with two fingers, and replaced the wallet. Then he ran off. I preferred not to do anything. The guy often does this to other people. I don't know if he carries a weapon.

These places were so dangerous that one method of protection was to always go with two or more friends.

Similarly, there was also a danger of being mugged in the movie theaters and we heard stories about this, mainly involving people who were new to these places. A very experienced client told the ethnographer about a friend of his who went to the movies very well dressed and wearing valuable jewelry, some time ago. He was mugged in the toilets by two men who threatened him with a knife. They stole everything from him and left him in his underpants. The man who told the story had to go to the victim's house and bring him some clothes. The victim stopped going to the movie theater for a while, though he has since returned. Now he wears less trendy clothes.

According to Victor:

> I heard about muggings. A queen who's a friend of mine told me he was mugged by two gay guys in the bathroom. At first they let him suck them. He was doing it when he felt a blow on the back of his neck. It wasn't so hard because he reacted immediately. They grabbed him by the neck and mugged him. They stole his chains and his money.

LOCUSTS

By 1998, crime had not diminished. In fact, it had increased sharply. More than twenty-five gay men have been murdered in recent years. Many *cacheros* and gay sex workers have also been mugged and attacked by criminals. Nevertheless, this continuous pattern of violence cannot blind us or obscure the significant changes that have taken place in public sex places. One of these is the appearance of the *chapulines* or locusts. They are so-called because people liken them to the swarming pests that attack crops. Locusts are juvenile gang members who mug and rob people. However, instead of invading the countryside, their sphere of action is the city. They operate in groups, and while one immobilizes the victim in an armlock, the rest rob him of his belongings. Sometimes, "immobilize" means stab with a knife. The locusts are both male and female, but here we are only concerned with the former, because they are the ones who have sexual relations with gays.

The locusts are a focus of attention in this study because they are the group that is most antagonistic toward gays in public places, and because they are responsible for the majority of the murders of gay men that have occurred in recent years. They, like the gays, have been taking over public places to impose their own culture. Their appearance in Costa Rican society dates back to about ten years ago, approximately the same time as the upsurge in public sex places.

Eight years ago, there was a division of labor between *cacheros* or prostitutes, and criminals. The first made money from gays in exchange for sex. The second robbed both gays and prostitutes. The criminals were thieves, pure and simple. Their objective was to rob people, nothing more. On a few rare occasions they would make certain sexual advances to trick their victims. But they would eschew all sexual contact with them.

By 1998, things had changed significantly. The main criminals were now the locusts, who had driven out and displaced the traditional hoodlums. By operating in gangs, they had developed a whole new street culture. When asked about their identity, they proudly describe themselves as *chapulines*, a way of life. The development of their awareness of themselves as a minority merits a separate book. However, what concerns us in this study is that the locusts are significantly different from the old-style criminals and the traditional *cacheros*. They have evolved toward a combination of sex, robbery, and death. At some imprecise moment during the past few years, the locusts ceased to be mere delinquents and became part-time *cacheros*. In other words, many of them stopped mugging gays and began to fuck them *and* rob them, a lethal combination.

The question that comes to mind is, what happened during these years to trigger this change among the locusts and what is it about their culture that poses such an enormous threat to their homosexual clients?

THE VULNERABLE BODY

Locusts, along with many juvenile delinquents who prostitute themselves,[8] share a common history of abuse and violence at home. From all the interviews carried out with participants in the El Salon project,[9] both *cacheros* and locusts, we find that abuse was common. As children, they experienced all types of punishment and cruelty. They were raised by people who vented their rage against them using tape recorder cables (Alberto), rods (David), whips made from dried squash vines (Antonio), hoses filled with sand (Heriberto), electric cables (Josué), and punches, floggings, and stones (Mario). Some lived with mothers who were prostitutes or with fathers who abused them sexually (Deni, Rolando). Mario's case stands out, though it is not unusual:

> My dad was an alcoholic and took money from my mom to pay for his booze. Since he didn't work, if my mother didn't give him money he would beat her and beat us too. One day he grabbed her and began punching her and forced her to open her mouth. She begged him: "No! You can't leave me without my false teeth!" Well, the sonofabitch beat her, forced her mouth open, pulled out her false teeth, and sold them for a bottle.

Why so much violence? When we asked them why they were beaten so much, they could not find a reason; they just stared blankly. They grew up in homes which had no future for them. The locust from the smallest family had seven siblings and the one from the largest had eighteen. These large families were the result of the Catholic church's antifamily planning policy. The people who raised these children lost their patience easily and quickly. There was no way to maintain so many children, and money and work were harder to come by every day. It was their fathers, stepfathers, or the companions of their mothers who were the most sadistic and brutal. These jobless men, who were addicted to drugs and alcohol, imposed their power physically. No longer able to provide food regularly for their families, they maintained their macho privileges through violence. Thus, the locusts' school of violence is closely related to gender issues: it serves to preserve gender imbalances. This phenomenon is important to understand why locusts use so much violence against their clients when gender rules are disregarded.

At some point in time, the future locusts began their own revolution of the body: escape from home. There was no food and no structure for them. Families disintegrated. "We all went our own way," says Girasol. Most ran away from their homes before the age of ten. With one or two exceptions, none of the interviewees had a home. They had been thrown out by their parents or had fled from their homes and now live on the streets, in slums or drug addicts' "bunkers." "More than twenty of us [locusts] live in this park," says Guillermo. "When it rains, we get wet. Everyone grabs a bench for a bed. If the cops come around, we ask them what's the point of moving us if we have no place to go?" It goes without saying that they make a living from robbery, the sex trade, and drugs. The pattern is the same as the one Russel found in his study on male prostitutes in the United States. According to Russel, one of the main factors to explain prostitution and drug addiction was "the absence of support in homes replete with children, from which the future prostitutes were thrown out onto the street to fend for themselves."[10] To survive, as MacNamara tells us in his analysis of male prostitution in American cities, they sell their bodies, the only salable thing they have.[11] However, Snell does not find the same pattern among the street prostitutes in his study: unlike Costa Rica's locusts, only 10 percent of the young men who prostitute themselves in the public places of the U.S. capital actually live on the streets.[12]

Most locusts were subjected to a kind of violence that inured them to the penetration of their bodies by ferocious and inept parents or guardians. No punishment could be accepted as rational when they did not even have food or a place to live. The slums could not cope with so many children, and every new arrival displaced the previous child. When these kids fled, they promised themselves that nobody would ever lay a finger on them again. "No sonofabitch is going to lay a hand on me again," says Guillermo. "I've already had enough, so I couldn't take another blow." Luis shares this view: "Nobody touches me unless I want them to. Nobody who wants to stay alive."

In the streets the locusts acquired a great knowledge of the weaknesses of Latin American cities. To become experts in urban guerilla warfare, it was necessary to study the different areas of the city and the minds of its inhabitants. Open public spaces were identified as being most vulnerable: parks, commercial centers, movie theaters, toilets, and recreation centers. At the same time, victims were targeted if they appeared distracted: a woman window-shopping, a young man enjoying himself with his girlfriend, a pair of lovers at the movies or on a dark road, an office worker in a hurry. All would be easy prey for these young men by being in public places and letting their minds wander. While the woman gazed at the store window and wondered what that blouse might look like on her, or the young man kissed his girlfriend and closed his eyes to enhance the feeling, the locusts would pounce on them and steal their belongings.

Their interest in the open and vulnerable places in cities and for the people in them would lead the locusts to share a very particular vision of the body and sexuality. Like the marginal social groups to which they belong, locusts believe that gender and sexuality are inscribed in the body. However, it is a body which is seen as a battlefield. Just as a city has open and attractive spaces for the public, so too does the body. The difference between victim and aggressor lies in the ability to open and close these spaces. The locusts are obsessed with orifices. Theirs must remain closed to the world; those belonging to others are ready to be taken.

When sexuality is centered in the body and not in the mind, or in some invisible ethereal personality, homosexuality is determined by the organs and their functions. For a locust, a homosexual is someone who allows his body to be invaded. Although homosexuality can be inherited and people can be born homosexual, practice can also lead the body toward a "sexual inversion." In this respect, their views are no different from the nineteenth-century doctors who, as Margaret Gibson points out, believed that homosexuality was inscribed in the body but, like the plague, could be acquired through practice.[13] Locusts believe in hereditary factors but also in the notion of a vulnerable body. Nobody should let his guard down, because at any moment danger can strike: like a virus, homosexuality can invade.

Homosexual orientation is, then, an invaded orifice. Anyone can suffer this invasion: we all have orifices. When this occurs, the organs themselves are transformed and become "homosexualized."

"That queen I screw is dominated by her ass. She has an insatiable faggot ass. She's lost control of her own asshole." "And yours?" we ask José, a locust. "What is your ass like?" "Mine is a man's ass," he replies proudly. "I've trained it only to *shit*!" "It seems like you're talking about a pet and not about a part of yourself," we remark. "Yeah, the ass is like a dog. You have to kick it so it understands that it should only follow its master," he concludes.

LITTLE PINK RIDING HOOD CONFRONTS THE BIG BAD WOLF

It is probable that the encounter between gays and locusts was something that nobody wanted or expected. Unlike the *cacheros*, locusts did not have contact with homosexuals that stretched back to time immemorial. *Cacheros* have long had relations with gays in prisons, on ships in the navy, on police forces, and in all Latin places where women were scarce. Among the lower classes, men may penetrate other men when there are no women or when there is a lot of liquor around, without suffering the stigma of homosexuality. A common joke in Costa Rica asks: what is the difference between a homosexual man and a Latin heterosexual? The answer: three beers inside.

But the gangs of *chapulines* have enough *chapulinas*—female gang members—and therefore cannot be compared with sailors, prison inmates, banana workers, or truck drivers, who spend much of their time away from women. There must have been another reason for them to copy some of the patterns of these groups. The only one we can find in their stories is that the relationship developed through sharing the same physical spaces. Locusts and gays invaded the same public spaces, during the same decade, for different reasons. The encounter was inevitable as the parks, public toilets, movie theaters, and public pools became their homes.

But this does not explain why the locusts went from being muggers to *cacheros*. What did they find in these common spaces that would lead them to go beyond the earlier criminals? This is a key question, because it explains, in part, why they became killers of homosexuals.

THE LOOK: FROM CHAPULINES *TO PRINCES*

The *chapulines* cannot recall the exact moment when they became sex workers. At some imprecise time in their lives, they went from being criminals to being criminals who do sex work. The only common denominator in their histories is the recollection that, in some public place, a homosexual turned to look at them. The recollection of that first look is what still remains in their heads, which are now filled with crack and glue and are not altogether clear:

> All I can remember is being in Parque Pinochet ready to mug a guy and take his chain. Suddenly, I see this guy watching me, kind of shadowing me. The guy makes me nervous. "Why's that shithead looking at me? Is he a cop?" I think to myself. But I know how to recognize a cop. You see the look of hatred in their eyes. This guy wasn't looking at me with hate. But I didn't understand why he was watching me. It bothered me and it screwed up my hit [robbery]. (Miguel)

> To be a successful locust you must be inconspicuous. In other words, people shouldn't notice you. You do your work when they're distracted. But when someone is watching what you do, everything gets complicated and there's no privacy to do a good hit. This started happening to me in Parque Monumental. When I noticed that some people were watching me, I got upset. (Armando)

Deciphering the meaning and desire in another person's gaze takes time. It produces intrigue and curiosity, but also confusion. "I didn't understand," says José, "why they stared at my cock. Nobody had ever looked at me that way before. Is there something weird about my dick?" I wondered. Ernesto was surprised when he noticed men gazing into his eyes. "Women would tell me that I had nice eyes, but what did guys see in them?"

The gaze and observation of the gays had an impact on the criminal culture. Their supposed invisibility to citizens with distracted minds was coming to an end. Yet another actor was entering the scene of the crime. What would his role be? Would he talk to the police? Would he help the victims or not?

But this would not be the most important impact of the gays' interest in the locusts. There were two things in their observation that differed from the locusts' experience to date: attention and desire. The gaze of these experts in male beauty revealed something that the locusts had never suspected: that some of them were attractive young men. What the women of their class never even dreamed of, the gays had the imagination to see: inside this dirty, ragged toad was a handsome prince. All that was missing was a way of breaking the spell.

A fairy tale began because of that gaze: the public places bewitched their inhabitants.

> I don't know when I began to whore, but I do recall that I found I could make 5,000 colones by just taking out my dick and letting some queen suck it. It had never occurred to me that people would pay so much just because it was big. But word spread through the park that I had a big cock and my clientele increased. One night I made 50,000 colones by just letting people suck it. That's a lot better than risking jail for stealing someone's neck chain! (Luis)

> I discovered that my body was a good business. When I walk through the park, men turn to look at me. I know I provoke sexual desire in them. Some tell me I'm a really gorgeous guy. It hadn't even occurred to me. When I arrive, the guys fight each other to get my attention. (Horacio)

> I have a big butt. When I walk, the guys watch me with desire. I can even feel their gaze warming my ass. (Pedro)

Attractive, well-endowed locusts would find new benefits. As in any meat market, good "cuts" are the most appetizing and obviously the most expensive. This new money influenced the social differences that evolved within the locust community. Previously, the fastest and most aggressive individuals were the most powerful, the gang leaders. Now a new class was emerging: the handsome *chapulines* with big dicks and big asses. Those who did not satisfy the demands of the market remained as intermediaries of the "good beef":

> I told my partner in crime the truth: "You don't have a great dick and you have an ugly face. You're better off promoting

mine and I'll give you a commission. So, while I screw a client, you go find me some more." The guy accepted 500 colones for each client.

> Not all *chapulines* are pretty. Some can earn money because they're macho-looking, but generally it's us pretty guys who make all the money. I have plenty of clients because they say I look like a movie star. (Angel)

The attention of the gays led to the emergence of a new class of locusts and created a kind of magic in parks and public places. For a few hours, undocumented delinquents, drug-addicts, and criminals, who were despised and feared by decent people, became public porn stars. A new Cinderella was born. The new heroes of this fairy tale no longer had to sweep and clean out their victims: now they could fuck them and make good money off them:

> I don't deny that I like the attention. I go to the park now and I know that people say: "Here comes that delicious guy." When I go walking, men follow me all over the place. I feel like the king of the dicks. Although I don't like guys, I do like it when these rich shitheads look for me and beg me to give it to them up their ass. I like to see them humiliate themselves. (Horacio)

> I don't understand why they like to suck dick so much. When I take it out in the park, they even line up. One day, I let six of them do it. I charged them 500 colones each for just two minutes a turn. I even had to scold them and tell them to line up so they'd all get a turn. I've even thought of handing out numbered tokens so there won't be so much disorder. (Fabricio)

> This is good business. Last week, two guys wanted me to go with them. One offered me 7,000 and the other 8,000. The first just wanted to suck me. The second wanted me to fuck him. We were discussing the deal when a third came up and offered me 10,000 to spend the whole night. "What do you want me to do?" I asked. "Well, I like to watch porn and you can rub my dick," he suggested. So then I said to the three of them, "What if the four of us go off together and I'll do to each one what-

ever he wants, and you pay me 25,000 between the three of you. "No, no!" one of the clients said. "Everything for 20,000." So I agreed to give them a discount. (Pedro)

The new locust class involved in prostitution also began to "invest" in their small businesses:

> Here you need to fix yourself and dress well to get clients. You can be poor but you must be clean and smell good. I bathe here, in El Salon, and buy myself a nice little shirt to go to the movies or the park. I also got rid of the tangles in my hair and got myself a new haircut. (Horacio)

> If you want to make money in this business you have to know how to present yourself better. My trick is to buy old faded jeans and wear them without underpants. That way clients can see shapes and sizes. If you don't wear underpants, the heat fades the jeans and you can see the size perfectly. That way you can charge more and people can see the goods. (Fabricio)

> I always carry a little bottle of scent. When someone sucks me, they leave their odor on my body. With a little perfume, I'm ready for the next one without them noticing that I've already been with someone. (Ricardo)

But every fairy tale has its problems. At some point, the spell that transforms a horrible and sad reality into a dream comes to an end. Princes turn back into frogs and the queens return to their castles in the middle-class suburbs of San José. The man who yesterday fought to conquer the chapuline of his life returns to his job and forgets about him. The one who surrendered his body in a frenzy of passion now crosses the street when they meet in downtown San José. However, things can never be the same again. Cinderella has seen the castle and has tasted the elixir that transported her to an unimaginable world: now she knows how things might have been if she had been born in the castle. She also feels she has a certain value she never had before: we could say that her self-esteem has grown. But is it necessary to commit crimes for this?

Chapter 8

Clash of Cultures

Though they may have the best of sex, locusts and gays inhabit totally different planets. For gays, with their sexual model of the body and its pleasures, and locusts with their vision of the vulnerable body, communication is a tortuous road. The same words do not have the same meanings; nor do certain practices mean the same things. A simple desire, the slightest touch to the body, can unleash chaos. One moment someone might be taking a man to the point of orgasm, and the next to the point of death. In seconds, a torrid passion can turn into a bloodbath. Love can turn to anger. A term of endearment can be perceived as the greatest of insults. If some spoke Chinese and the others Russian there might be fewer problems. Things become more dangerous when we think we are speaking the same language, but in fact are not.

An example of this is the wave of homosexual murders in the past few years. Approximately twenty-five gay men have been the victims of *cacheros* and some have been killed by locusts. These crimes go beyond simple robbery. They are forms of torture that are impregnated with an unusual degree of rage.

A typical case was the murder of Klaus, a man in his forties, who was found dead in the capital at a hotel used exclusively for sex. According to his friend Luis, Klaus had received thirty-five stab wounds all over his body. His rectum had been cut into several pieces and so had his tongue. His penis was found in a vase. There was so much blood in the bed that a bucket was needed to gather it up. The walls were also spattered with blood: Klaus had put up a real fight for his life. Bloodstains from his assailants were found all over the room. Several jugs and glasses were smashed. Some bore Klaus' fingerprints—he had probably tried to defend himself with them. Although he had screamed for help, his cries were drowned out by loud music. The police believe Klaus struggled with his attackers for about ten minutes before collapsing on the floor dead. The multiple stab wounds must have weakened him until he could no longer go on. Aside from the victim, at least two more men were in the room. The killers still have not been found.

Another victim was Eduardo. According to Hector, his friend and confidant, this forty-one-year-old gay man lived alone in a condominium in the south of San José. Opposite the door of his second-floor apartment lived Clotilde, a woman friend. Although Clotilde would get upset at Eduardo for allowing all types of men into the building, she would always be sure to peer out to see who came to visit him. One night she heard the doorbell ring when three men arrived. Eduardo opened the door and invited them in. A few minutes later, Clotilde heard the stereo system being turned on. "Oh, no!" she thought to herself. "I wonder how late they're going to be up making noise," she said to her husband. "It's none of your business," he replied. Both knew Eduardo was gay and they had a good relationship with him. Aside from inviting his friends over, he would help them in any way he could and would take care of their apartment whenever they were out of town. They even had a key to his apartment. However, a few minutes later the volume was turned way up. "Alvaro, something's wrong," Clotilde said to her husband.

Clotilde saw the three men leave the apartment with a large bag. They seemed agitated and in a hurry. One of them was looking all around, as if wishing to make sure that they had not been seen. She closed the drapes to avoid being seen. Intrigued, she convinced her husband to ring Eduardo's doorbell. "Ask him if he needs anything," she said anxiously. Alvaro rang the doorbell, but there was no reply. He waited a minute and then tried again. "Clotilde, there's no answer. Go get the key to his apartment," he told his wife. Clotilde ran to find the key. She wondered where she might have put it. Eduardo had given her the key more than a year ago, just in case of an emergency, and she had never used it. At last she found it in one of the drawers in her bedroom. The minutes spent searching for the key still haunt her. "If we'd gotten to him more quickly, perhaps we could have done something," she told us.

When the couple entered Eduardo's apartment there was total chaos. Not a single thing was in its place. "How could they break so much in such a short time?" they both wondered. They ran to the bedroom and opened the door. Clotilde describes what she saw:

> There was blood all over the bedroom. When I looked at the bed, I saw Eduardo totally amputated: no arms and no penis. My God! I screamed like a crazy woman. Only the torso was in one piece. The flesh on his arms and legs hung from the bones. He was still alive and just had time to say: "My friends killed me. Tell my mom I love her very much," and he fell dead on the floor.

Clotilde began to scream and tried to help her neighbor. However, her husband realized that nothing could be done:

> Clotilde was in a state of hysteria. When she tried to lift him, she ended up with a piece of flesh in her hands. He had so many knife wounds that he looked like a sieve. I made her leave the room and told her to call the police. When they came they told me that Eduardo had twelve stab wounds in his rectum and that they had not only cut off his arms but even a leg.

The case of Julio, age forty-nine, was similar. His former lover told us that the last time he was seen alive was at 9:30 on a Friday night when he let three men into his apartment. Some other gay men lived downstairs and they had visitors that night. The loud music prevented them from hearing anything of what happened upstairs. Julio was found the following day by his ex-lover:

> Julio's sister called me. She was very worried because he hadn't shown up at his nephew's christening. She asked me to go check that he was okay. I told her not to worry, that I would go over immediately. When I entered his apartment, I saw that he'd been robbed. Everything was a mess: the drawers were open, the sound system had gone, and the decorations were all broken. However, I didn't see Julio. I looked for him everywhere, including his bedroom. There was a bundle of clothes

on the bed but no sign of him. I decided to use the phone that was on the night table to call the police, and moved the sheets to sit down on the bed. Horror of horrors! As I pulled back the sheets I noticed that Julio was underneath. He was dead. One sheet was stuffed into his throat. He had been asphyxiated and tortured. The police told me later that they found both his testicles in his throat. His buttocks had been burned with cigarettes.

THE LANGUAGE OF CRIME

In an attempt to understand the criminal mentality we searched for studies on homophobes who kill gay men. Martin Kantor has devised the most elaborate classification of the different types of criminals.[1] According to this author, the type of crime we are dealing with here involves killers with "emotional disorders." Kantor believes these are generally men who have low self-esteem and who feel their lives have no meaning. When they compare themselves with gays they generally feel great envy and a desire to destroy them to prove to themselves that nobody should be above them, much less men who belong to a minority. The author believes that this type of homophobe is paranoid because he projects an exaggerated sense of well-being toward his enemies.[2]

Although the envy and rage that locusts feel toward gays is similar to that felt by the blue-collar workers studied by Kantor, it would be unfair to label them paranoid: the truth is, they do have a point. "What do you mean we *imagine* that homosexuals have everything that we don't have?" asks Girasol. "The truth is, they *do*." Moreover, the locusts seek out the gays just as much as the gays seek them. Unlike the North American blue-collar workers who seek out homosexuals to attack them physically (gay bashing), the locusts are as much the pursued as the pursuers. "We don't go around looking for gays to screw them. They look for us," says Pepe.

To understand and prevent such horrible murders, we decided it would be best to ask the locusts themselves to explain these crimes. After all, they are the experts on the subject. With the cooperation of the director of the El Salon program, we selected ten *chapulines* who are sex workers and who have been on the point of killing—or have actually killed—a gay client or *pagador* as they call them. First, we described the previously mentioned crimes to them (some knew the victims and the aggressors) and asked them to give us a "reading" or interpretation of the murder script.[3]

Most of the locusts interviewed agreed that the motive in all three cases was robbery. "It's obvious that the guys wanted to rob them," says Girasol. "Two or three *chapulines* probably got together and went to visit an old client. He probably fucked with one of them and trusted him enough to let him in with the others," he continues. "The biggest mistake," says Pepe, "is to let more than one guy in the house. When locusts go around in a group it means they're planning a hit. We would never fuck in front of our buddies," he says. "But why did they decide to kill this guy if one of them had fucked with him?" we ask. "Because a locust won't kill the first time. He needs to study the place, the person, his habits in order to then do the hit. Often years go by before he can do it," explains Gerardo. "Probably the gay was being cheap and wouldn't hand over the dough," adds Carlitos. Eduardo thinks that there might have been an argument: "Those three guys who were killed in a row were all drunks and bad-mouths, queens with poisonous tongues. Perhaps they insulted a locust or tried to some weird thing," he adds.

"If they were only going to mug them or rob them, why kill them and mutilate their bodies?" we ask. Julio believes that these crimes occur when the locusts have taken a combination of drugs: crack, marijuana, and alcohol. "Anything that makes you crazy. Probably they were all stoned and then they had an argument over money and they went wild and began to attack. Once you begin, you can't stop." Girasol, on the contrary, believes it was all premeditated. "The fact that three of them showed up means they were going to rob him. They had it all figured out," he says with confidence.

There is a greater degree of consensus with respect to the mutilations: all three victims had their orifices filled. "The three were stabbed in the ass, the mouth, and the dick," says José. "This means the locusts wanted to punish them for being gays, for letting themselves be fucked." Girasol agrees. "We can't understand how a man would want someone to put a dick up his ass or in his mouth. It's not natural. Even the priests won't forgive you for that. I think these guys wanted to send a message that these gays were sick and that's why they killed them," he says. Pepe, however, believes that the severed hands might indicate that the client touched the locust on his private parts in an improper way. A severed penis suggests that the client had taken advantage of circumstances and had possessed him previously. This excessive violence is related to the kind of abuse the locusts experienced as children: those who do not respect the rules of gender are punished. Just as they saw their fathers put their mothers "in their place" when the latter would not give them money for liquor, so they punish the *pagadores* who do things that are not proper for men or who refuse to pay them the money they want.

We then asked the interviewees to give us a list of "triggers" that might make someone move from sex to crime. Since the locusts had not forced their way into any of their victims' homes, we were intrigued to know what factors might have lit the fuse. It was clear that this was not the first time they had interacted with their victims. In some cases, the victims were regular clients of the locusts. Others, such as Klaus, had sex with more than 1,000 locusts before meeting their deaths at the hands of three of them. What could make the difference between having sex one night and killing the next? The *chapulines* gave us a long list of "triggers."

TRIGGERS TO **CHAPULINE** *VIOLENCE*

Not Respecting the Agreed Price or Asking for Unjustified Discounts

Among locusts there is an almost unanimous belief that many gays agree to pay a given sum and then try to cheat them. They also agree that this is the main cause of violent attacks. Juan José nearly killed a gay who made him take out his penis to masturbate him in a park and then fled without paying him the 3,000 colones he had been promised. Luis attacked a man with a bottle when the client, who had offered him 5,000 colones to penetrate him, and done so, claimed he only had 3,000. Mikol was furious when he agreed to give a discount to a client who said he only had 2,000 colones and, when he pulled down his pants and the wallet fell out by accident, Mikol saw that it contained more than 20,000. He immediately took out a knife, stabbed him, and ran off with the money. Pepe was invited to an orgy at an apartment. After having engaged in sex with three gays, they offered him some old clothes. He immediately picked up the fish tank and smashed it over the host's head. He was so enraged that he couldn't contain himself and the victim ended up in intensive care. In other cases, clients pay the agreed sum but flaunt their wealth: they take the locusts to their luxurious homes or carry a lot of money around. Faced with such extravagance, any agreed price seems ridiculous to the locusts and an assault is imminent. Their addiction to crack also increases their need for money. All sexual activity is seen as a prelude to smoking one or two hits of crack. If the money does not materialize, their rage is enormous. "Look, you feel hungry and haven't eaten for a day. A client comes up and offers you 5,000 for a fuck. You work out the numbers and see yourself smoking some crack. If the guy doesn't pay up, you feel like killing him and sometimes you do it," Girasol confesses.

Humiliation

Chapulines believe that many gays despise them and treat them without respect. Carlos, for instance, tells us that he was enraged when one of his clients complained about the size of his penis. At that moment, he took out his knife and stabbed the gay man. "Nobody makes fun of my size and lives to tell the story," he says. Others make them feel bad by complaining about their odor. Juan Antonio punched a client who he told him he couldn't stand the smell of his feet. "The sonofabitch didn't care that I shoved my dick all the way up him in the park, but at his house he complained about my feet," he tells us. "I shoved a knife in his ass so he would stop complaining about the smell." Luis went to eat at a Chinese restaurant with his client after making love in the park. "The guy complained about the way I ate my soup," he tells us angrily. "I grabbed the hot soup and threw it in his face, so he'll learn to keep his mouth shut," he says with satisfaction.

Disregard for Roles

We have seen how locusts share the idea that homosexuality is a form of behavior inscribed in the body. People become homosexuals because they change the masculine and aggressive role of the male. Thus, "male men," as they call themselves, are then ones who are not penetrated and who don't do "women's things." Doing "women's things" means kissing, allowing oneself to be penetrated, and giving oral sex. When a client tries to penetrate them or touches them in an "improper" way, he is severely punished. "This guy tried to fuck me. I'd already made it real clear that I'm a macho man and never give my ass. When we went to his apartment, he tried to rape me. I grabbed my knife and stuck it into his stomach. No sonofabitch touches my ass!" Pedro assures us. With the crack boom, some locusts admit that they have been forced to "give their ass" and "do things one doesn't want to do" because they are desperate for money. Although in theory they do so voluntarily, they feel a tremendous rage at having to abandon their principles. At any moment, a small spark can ignite the fire. "That sonofabitch forced me to suck him for six reds [6,000 colones]. When the guy fell asleep, I put some gas on his ass and lit him up," says Pepe.

What does changing roles mean for the locusts? It is not always easy to guess. For some *chapulines*, being asked to wash dishes in an apartment or to help in the kitchen may be seen as an attempt to feminize them. Carlitos nearly punched his client in the mouth when he was asked to help him chop onions. "That bastard wanted to treat me like a broad," he recalls. "If he wants a maid, he should get a woman," he says. Another way of making them feel as if they are being feminized is to be taken to gay bars or homosexual meetings. June broke two of his client's teeth when, without permission, he invited three gay friends of his to meet June: "That asshole wanted to sweet-talk me and introduce me as his husband," he says.

Poor Labor Relations

For the locusts, clients are a source of income. Unlike gays, sexual pleasure is totally irrelevant to them. The majority are heterosexual and do not enjoy sex with men. When a client or *pagador* establishes a relationship with a locust, the latter expects some form of compensation when the relationship is broken off. For the criminal, there is no justification for ending a relationship for passionate or amorous reasons. Juan killed Victor when, after three years of being his client, Victor found himself another locust. Gerardo cut off one of his client's testicles when he found out that he was paying another *chapuline* more than him. In the case of Ricardo, when he realized that his client had decided to live with another locust, he set fire to his apartment "with the queen and everything inside," he admits.

Homophobia

Most locusts, as Fernando tells us, "hate queens." This means that they share society's feelings of contempt toward homosexuals. To have to depend on them in order to eat or to buy drugs creates a permanent hostility. Since locusts do not consider themselves as homosexuals or enjoy sex with men, they are probably more intolerant. (It would be necessary to analyze the difference between *cachero* prostitutes and locusts in a subsequent study to evaluate sexual pleasure, or its absence, as a factor in violence against gays.)

When a gay, in the eyes of a locust, behaves in a very feminine way or draws attention to himself in the street, he does so to "humiliate me" (the locust). If the gay is sexually passive, the locusts despise him for allowing himself to be penetrated. On some occasions, generally when they have taken a mixture of drugs, any "weird move," as they term a mannerism, can provoke an attack. According to Carlitos, when he fucks a gay and sees him being feminine and content with his passivity, "I want to grab him by the balls to make him into a man." Once, when he had smoked some crack, he began to beat a client with a club. According to the locusts, the most dangerous time to provoke a homophobic attack is the moment after ejaculation. "When I come, I feel this enormous rage about needing to have sex for money. At that moment," confesses Pedro, "I feel like killing the client. I feel disgusted and it makes me mad. I'll turn any one of them into pulp."

Finally we asked the locusts to put themselves in the place of their clients. What advice would they give them to help them avoid being killed by *chapulines*? The following was the list they gave us.

TEN RULES THAT COULD SAVE LIVES

1. It is better to have sex in public places than at home. Locusts have fewer opportunities to kill a client in public places. They might mug him, but they will only be able to take what he is carrying, instead of everything he owns. Clients should not agree to go to another "more private" place—in other words, a deserted place. Other people are their protection.
2. Never flaunt your wealth or wear fine clothes or jewelry. This is what provokes most anger among people who have nothing. It is best to take only enough money to pay for sex. Do not use your car as a motel or allow anyone to get inside it.
3. Always pay the agreed sum. Do not try to negotiate after sex or make changes to the agreement. Nor should you change the method of payment: locusts want cash.
4. Do not make advances or ask for things that were not agreed upon. Be especially careful about everything related to anal sex.
5. If you plan to invite a locust to your home, ask for his identity card and say you will write down the number and give it to a friend in case something bad happens. Inform your friends about these visits.
6. Never let more than one locust into your house. When more than one shows up, it is because they are up to something. Nor you should let in a locust who has been sent by someone else. Even if you let only one into your house, he may have planned something with others waiting outside for an opportunity to strike.
7. Do not take drugs with locusts. Combination drugs are fatal and explosive. It will be harder to attack you if you are sober.
8. Keep a weapon that you can use. Locusts always carry knives or guns. However, be sure that you know how to fight. Many clients think they are more skilled than they really are. Locusts are expert fighters.
9. Do not argue with a locust. They have problems with verbal language and you will always win an argument. However, when it comes to body language and street language, you are at a disadvantage.

10. Never make comments about their smell or lack of education, much less their size or way of doing things.

A VISIT TO THE CASTLE

The gays' vision of sexuality is "modern," as opposed to that of the locusts. Gays believe that people's sexuality is determined by the object of desire. For gays, sexuality is an internal and fixed phenomenon that is not determined by practice. Whether one is active or passive, one can still be gay. For them, the body is not a battleground but a source of pleasure: both the orifices and the protruding organs form part of sexuality. Therefore, if they go to bed with men, they do not see the need to protect themselves like a fortress. Femininity and masculinity are not regarded as permanent and rigid structures, but as characteristics that change in time and space. If yesterday men could not cook, today they can do so and it is not the end of the world. What was masculine yesterday might not be today. If a gay man prepares a dinner for his partner, the latter is not feminized because he has to wash the dishes.

This model clashes with that of the locusts. For these two groups, each word acquires a different meaning. For gays, a homosexual and a locust who goes to bed with men are one and the same thing. Sex workers are often termed gays. If you are going to have sex with another man, the gays believe that both bodies are there to be touched and enjoyed. For them, homosexuality does not reside in the backside, nor is it governed by hormones or chemical substances. They cannot understand how a locust can consider the rectum to be the sacred altar of masculinity, the forbidden city of the body. Thus, when they become better acquainted with a locust, they will try to fondle him there, believing that if he does not enjoy it is because he is a frustrated homosexual. It goes without saying that this leads gays to commit errors of judgment which the locusts resent.

However, if the problem were simply a matter of linguistics, "*Cachero*-Gay—Gay-*Cachero*" dictionary would resolve the conflict. In this hypothetical dictionary we would find, for example, the following explanations:

	***Cachero*-Gay Dictionary**	**Gay-*Cachero* Dictionary**
Homosexual	man who allows himself to be penetrated	person who has sex with someone of the same sex
Queen	woman in a man's body	any gay that we don't like
Man	a male who fucks everyone	butch queen
Woman	delicate and passive individual	a being represented by transvestites
Client	all queens	old queen
Cachero	macho man	frustrated queen
Male	active man	a man before he drinks three beers
Backside	restricted access zone	leisure park
Penis	weapon to dominate the weak	typical food
Public places	home	first liberated territories of the Gay Republic

But even with such a dictionary, the misunderstandings would continue. Both groups share a territory that serves as a common link—for some to realize their fantasies and others to make money. So long as the territory is a public place, the magic spell seems to have the desired effect: the number of killings in these places is minimal. It is when people make the mistake of leaving public places for private spaces that killings take place, one after another.

One reason for this is that by leaving the parks, movie theaters, or toilets, the locusts and the gays see each other the way they did before coming under the magic spell, which, for a few brief moments, made them forget about class differences. On leaving Sexland, the cruel reality becomes evident: some are the favored and others are the oppressed. Let us consider the story of Joselito, a twenty-one-year-old locust, who was taken to a gay man's apartment:

> I was sitting on a bench one night in Colombia Park. I was hungry and cold. It was nighttime, around midnight. I hadn't picked up any clients and was fed up with waiting. Suddenly, a guy came up and sat next to me. He asked me if I was alone and what was I doing. I told him I was waiting for a friend. I

> noticed that the guy was staring at me. "You like me?" I asked. "Sure, you look real good," he said. I smiled so he would see I was interested. He was an old guy of about fifty. He asked if I wanted to go with him. I said that if I went, I would charge 5,000 colones and that I only liked being the man. I saw that the guy didn't object. "Well, you understand what I'm saying?" I asked him. "Sure I understand. But don't you think I'm kind of old for that? After all, you're just a kid. How can you do it to me?" he asked. "Well, only you can say whether or not you want me to do it to you. But I don't do anything else. And I don't suck either," I added. He told me he liked me so much that he was willing to do everything. We began walking and he told me his car was nearby. It just happened to be a BMW! I got in and we drove to his house. He lives in Rohrmoser [an expensive residential district of San José] in a huge mansion, and alone. When we arrived I saw a kind of luxury I'd never seen before in my life. The house was full of things everywhere. It looked like a museum. It made me so mad to see such luxury and me starving to death. "I have to rob this sonofabitch," I thought. Once we were in the bedroom, the guy asked me why I smelled so bad. He said I should go take a bath, that he wouldn't do anything if I didn't wash myself. At that moment I took out my knife and stuck it in his arm to frighten him. I grabbed everything I could and ran off.

We ask Joselito whether he would he have robbed and knifed his client if he had not been transported to a reality that would be better for him not to see. "I don't know what to say. If the old guy had given me his ass in the park and paid me five reds [5,000 colones], I wouldn't have done anything to him. But when he took me to his house and made me feel like scum, it made me mad," he tells us.

Let us now hear a client's viewpoint:

> Last year I went to Cinema 545. I sat in the back row where there were several men on their own. I noticed one who was masculine and blond, the kind I like. I moved and sat next to him and put my elbow on the armrest between us. He put his elbow there too and turned and smiled at me. For about ten minutes we didn't do anything but leave our elbows touching.

> I felt a tingling all over my body and the warmth of his arm. I liked the fact that the guy wasn't in a hurry. After a short time, which seemed like an eternity to me, he leaned over and gave me a delicious kiss. He said his name was Pablo and that he wanted to go with me. "Do you charge?" I asked discreetly. "Yes, but if you do what I want and do it well, I won't charge you anything," he said. I was totally confused, because I felt he was a very special person. By now I didn't care whether he charged or not. I invited him back home with me because my apartment is near the movie theater. When we went outside into the light, the guy looked haggard and badly dressed. Back at my apartment I noticed that he was spending a lot of time looking at my compact discs and my paintings. "How much did all these CDs cost you?" he asked. I tried to change the subject. However, I began to see the anger and the vulgarity in his face. When he took off his clothes, I saw that he was dirty—and he wanted me to give him oral sex! I must admit, I was very disgusted and asked him to leave. Fortunately, he didn't make a scene though I gave him 5,000 colones to avoid any problems. Later, I discovered that he'd stolen three CDs. I was so pissed! I wish I'd never left the movie theater.

This mutual deception is what leads clients to take a locust home. However, it is not too clear why some gays, as the locusts claim, take them home and do not pay them what they promise. One explanation might be that, as Esteban says, that "crooks never have a fixed price in mind. They try to see how much they can get. You pay them the agreed sum and they say that you promised them more. They want to see how much they can get out of you." This desire to modify the agreed price was also noted by MacNamara in his study of street prostitutes in New York City.[4] However, the *chapulines* themselves recognize that many of their transactions take place without a hitch and that only some are problematic. The fact that all the interviewees agree that clients sometimes try to cheat them suggests there is some truth in this.

One explanation of this phenomenon is rooted, possibly, in the disenchantment of the gays. In the model of bodies and pleasure, and in North American pornography, prostitution does not exist.

Porn movies never show the actors being paid or men buying sex. It is all deliciously voluntary. This is exactly how, in theory, sexual encounters should be in public places: good, beautiful, and free. But, after all the hard work of making contact, the torrid passion and living out a wonderful fantasy, an outstretched hand appears demanding money. It tells us that things were not what they seemed, that it was not a dream, and, worst of all to the ears of a persecuted minority: " I don't like you. What we did has a price." In the eyes of the prince, Cinderella once again turns into a simple employee, a ragged upstart. Now the gay client wants revenge, because Cinderella tricked him and didn't have education or class: "The fuck wasn't worth it. You don't know how to do things. Anyhow, how much do you want for that *shit* that we did?" says the client disparagingly.

The moment after ejaculation is the most dangerous of all. After the elixir that makes us forget that we live in an underdeveloped society, that princes will never marry "scum," and that these Cinderellas come to the ball to steal, sexual partners can become the worst enemies.

IS PUBLIC SEX REVOLUTIONARY?

Pat Califia considers public sex revolutionary in the United States.[5] The fact that people should rebel against thousands of years of Judeo-Christian sexual oppression and expose what ought to be hidden, because it is considered dirty and sinful, is one of the most important modern revolutions. She believes that "vanilla sex," or vaginal penetration—the only form of sexuality that is permitted—is a way of controlling men's and women's bodies. The author, who describes herself as a sadomasochist, believes that anything that challenges the established roles promotes a revolutionary fluidity that liberates people from patriarchal structures. With every whip lash on the backside of a male or female lover (she does not discriminate), the author sounds the trumpets that will bring down the walls of the Christian, middle-class Jericho. Every cock sucked in a public park, in a sauna, or at the movies is the first step toward the revolution of the sexual proletariat. Long live the Revolution!

But this author has forgotten to examine the issue of class. After all, in these postmodernist times in which class is discussed only in Cuba and North Korea, it would not appear to be an important factor. Nevertheless, just as "vanilla sex" represses the other forms of sex, so does middle-class sex repress those of the other social classes. In a society that is terribly divided by the accumulation of wealth, sucking a penis in a park does not have the same meaning for a middle-class gay man as it has for a half-starved locust. The act may seem the same. After all, how can there be a proletarian or bourgeois way of sucking a penis? But, as Derrida warns us, the meanings of language are "undeterminable": some suck heaven and others suck hell. That is why the philosopher used the word "Pharmakon" to refer to language: it can be medicine or poison.

Public sex in Latin America uses the language of pornography. During a few moments of pleasure, it seems that the terrible economic inequalities of developing nations have been erased. The ragged locust becomes a porn star, pursued by middle-class men who are educated, rich, and powerful. But once you ejaculate the spell is broken. Cinderella must return to the streets and wait for another client. The poor and miserable of this earth must return to their reality. The hand that reaches out and asks for money is always the same one in these countries. Is this revolutionary or is it the same exploitation and abuse that we already know?

Chapter 9

Police Officers

A third actor plays an important role in public places: the police officer.[1] His role is to ensure that such places are not used for sex or for criminal activities. Different police units patrol the places described. Part of the attraction of such places for gay men is the feeling of being at the mercy not just of criminals but also of the police. Sometimes the police officers arrest them or beat them up and sometimes they accept a bribe to let them go. Julio explains the role of the police in alleyways:

> One day I was walking toward the alley when someone I know stopped me and said it would be better if I didn't go near the place. He said there'd been a raid three days ago, so it was best to hang loose for a while. He said that on that day two patrol cars showed up and parked at each end of the alleyway. There were about fifteen guys in there and they couldn't move from the shock. Two minors were arrested because they didn't have ID cards; the rest were released, but they were trembling from fright. When something like that happens, people stay away from the alley for a few days.

Having sex in the park implies the possibility of being discovered. On some days, a patrol car will park on the north side of the park and remain there for several hours. From time to time, one or both officers get out of the car and stroll through the park, although the most usual procedure is for them to stay in the car. Gay men who frequent the park are aware of this, and have learned to communicate among themselves. When people who are in the darkest areas of the park start running away, the rest know there is trouble afoot.

"Run, boys, run, the cops are coming!" someone will hiss. In the southern sector of the park, the code used to warn others is to whistle a few bars of a song from the musical *West Side Story*. Whistling means that all sexual activity should stop. At that moment, gays and locusts generally call a truce and protect each other. The following dialogue, transcribed by one of our observers, is representative of what happens on such occasions. "How could you possibly say, officer, that we are queer?" says Ernesto, a locust. "My buddy," he adds, pointing toward the gay man, "came to the park so he could have a very serious discussion with me; we were discussing the rise in gasoline prices this week." "Sure!" the police officer replies. "I guess this little queen was lifting his tail to show how everything rises. Come on, I don't have time for jokes! Take out your ID or I'll arrest the two of you!"

Every day, between one and two in the morning, there is a changing of the guard at the embassies and public buildings in the surrounding area. The police officers, walking in pairs, march diagonally across Monument Park to the nearby police station. At that time, the park is practically empty. Once the changing of the guard has been completed, gay activities are resumed.

On one occasion when the area around Monument Park was in complete darkness and a lot of sexual activity was going on, the ethnographer watched as three patrol cars arrived. The police leaped out of their cars and turned on their flashlights. Very quickly, pairs of men could be seen scrambling away from the scene. In a few minutes, the park was deserted.

> The speed of the action was astonishing. I could see couples emerging from everywhere. They looked like cockroaches when you've sprayed the kitchen. A guy came running out holding his underpants in one hand. I suppose he put on his pants so quickly he forgot to put them on. Another guy was wearing his T-shirt inside out. A couple fell into a gutter. A locust took advantage of the situation to steal his client's sneakers. The other guy ran across the park in his socks.

Mario explains that people who are caught "in the act" are not always arrested:

> I didn't realize what was going on. . . . It was eleven at night. I was with some other guy. We were masturbating each other. The two of us had our pants down when we felt the flashlight on our faces. There was no time to do anything. Three cops approached us and asked us for our ID cards. Fortunately, the two of us were carrying our ID. Even so, they told us we were under arrest. I had a thousand colones with me. At one point I approached two of them and asked them if they would take my money instead of arresting us, and I was lucky: they let us go. Now, whenever I visit the park, I pay more attention.

The police also check on public toilets from time to time. According to Roberto:

> One night in November five guys and I were hanging out at this toilet, playing around with each other. It was about seven in the evening. All of a sudden, two cops appeared and made us leave. I was very scared. They made us stand against the wall and spread our arms and put our hands up against the wall. They also made us spread our legs and started to search us, like they do with criminals. I felt like I would die from shame, because at that time a lot of people were standing there waiting for the bus. When they finished searching us they let us go, after insulting us and calling us "corrupt." Those bastards did it on purpose, to embarrass us. I didn't go back there for two days, but now I go there later at night.

La Llanura Park is patrolled by mounted police officers. The officers in charge of policing this area say they arrest many couples:

> At night it's a gay carnival here. When you approach the parked cars, you see people masturbating each other or having oral sex. Homosexuals have become so cunning at throwing us off the track that they spread hay everywhere so the horses stop to eat and we can't catch them. The only thing they haven't done yet is bring mares in heat to distract our horses!

In the case of saunas and movie theaters, raids are less frequent since they are private businesses. However, the police have visited them on several occasions looking for minors or illegal aliens. Our ethnographer describes a police raid at the Sauna Laton:

> Mister, could you open up the door of your cubicle? We'd like to ask you a few questions. It's the police.
>
> Listen, redneck, I already told you I'm not gonna let you in. Can't you see I'm busy?
>
> Would you tell us what you're doing in that cubicle?
>
> Well, what the hell do you think I'm doing? I'm showing my Jacuzzi to a client.
>
> A what?
>
> I'm sucking someone off, asshole!
>
> Mister, you're under arrest. Come out so I can put the handcuffs on you.
>
> That's all I needed! An S and M queen!

THE TRAINED BODY

Costa Rican policemen tend to come from the poorer sectors of society. Many of them are from rural areas and moved to the city in search of better opportunities. They tend to come from large families. Our interviewees have many siblings. One of them lived with eighteen brothers and sisters: eleven from a first marriage, and seven from another. Their level of education is only marginally higher than that of the locusts. The majority have only attended primary school. A few went to high school but only a handful actually graduated. Their average salary is $200 a month, one of the lowest in the country.

In our in-depth interviews, we found a common denominator among policemen, gay men, and locusts: experience of physical violence during childhood. One of the policemen interviewed, Luis, used to get "the stick" (he was literally beaten with the branch of a tamarind tree) throughout his childhood and teenage years. Carlos was kicked so savagely by his mother that she broke his ribs on more than one occasion. Noé was so terrified of his stepfather's beatings that he spent a great deal of his childhood hiding under his bed. Miguel's older brother used to punch him in the face so badly he lost three teeth and often went around with split lips. "That's just what I remember," he adds. "I've forgotten a lot of what went on in those years." Sergio had to run away from home because of his grandfather's violence. "He was my real father. But he was an old-fashioned peasant, and he was very severe with us." When asked what "severe" means, he added, "He was strict. If you didn't work from four in the morning until ten at night, he would literally put your hands in the fire of the stove."

However, there are differences between policemen and locusts. Policemen generally do not come from broken homes. In spite of their poverty, they at least had one or two parents, or surrogate parents, to raise them. None of the twenty policemen interviewed had grown up on the street or in an orphanage. Therefore, they tend to display a certain gratitude and loyalty toward their caretakers. This makes it very difficult for them to consider such violence as a form of abuse, and they tend to defend their aggressors. Edwin, for instance, has this to say:

> They were very hard on me. However, I am thankful to them because they taught me to become a decent man, who likes things to be done properly. If they hadn't beaten me, I'd be in jail now, or I might be into drugs.

Aron feels the same way. He believes his parents behaved correctly when they punished him. "At the time I didn't understand why they belted me, but now I do. I was a very troublesome kid, and it was important that I should be raised properly." Benito thinks his father acted correctly when he used to punch him in the face. "He taught me never to say a four-letter word."

None of the interviewees protested against the physical violence they suffered as children. Apparently they accept the idea of violence as "education": the "spare the rod and spoil the child" syndrome, so to speak. The very middle-class and urban notion that children have rights and that they should not be subjected to excessive corporal punishment seems alien to them. When asked if they considered their caretakers' behavior to be inappropriate, the general response was "no."

However, the type of abuse they suffered at the hands of their parents or guardians seems to have been different from that suffered by the locusts. The actual violence may have been the same, but the motivation was different. The parents of the policemen used violence to "educate the body." In the case of locusts, as we have seen, violence was simply a way of imposing the power of gender.

Policemen's parents wanted their children to learn how to control their needs and desires. In a poverty-stricken society with large families, a child's life is harsh. Children are not "infants"; they are little adults. In rural zones, or marginal urban areas, children must contribute to the family income and help with household chores. Thus, domestic violence is directed at repressing childhood desires. The worst punishments are meted out when children want to do children's things: playing, going for a stroll, eating more than is allowed, or experimenting with their sexuality. According to José Alberto, there was never any time for such activities:

> The time I got my worst beating was when I ran away to swim in a pond. I'd been told to sweep the house and because I didn't do it, my dad grabbed a whip and gave me the worst lashing that I can remember.

These children were not allowed to say "obscenities," either. This concept embraces all common words related to sex. Not only did they never receive any sex education, their curiosity concerning sexual matters was actively repressed. Ernesto, a mounted police officer, lost a tooth after asking what "masturbation" meant.

> I'd heard the big word in school. In fact, I still find it hard to pronounce it. I went to my dad to ask him what it meant, and he punched me in the mouth. I lost a tooth. He told me, "Don't you ever come back to this house with dirty words again."

As children, most police officers learned that "the body is like a horse, which must be trained so you can mount it safely," as Fernando says (locusts tend to think of the body as a dog). A trained body, therefore, is one that has learned through punishment. Parents are the trainers; children, the trainees. A good child must learn to suppress desires that cannot possibly be satisfied in poor economic conditions. What is more, the child must not even express them.

Does a trauma exist when people are not even aware of it? The fact that police officers do not criticize their parents or caretakers does not mean that they have not suffered some kind of damage in their lives. Their sense of loyalty to their homes, their gratitude toward those who raised them, does not mean that the violence they experienced has been successfully resolved. There is much evidence to the contrary.

First of all, when we asked them if they raise their own children in the same way, they generally said no. Genaro, for example, told us that he does not spank his two children. "No, I don't think it's a good idea," he said. "But didn't you just say you thought it was good that you were punished as a child?" he was asked. "No, times have changed. Now it isn't good to do it," he replied. Aron agrees. "I've never spanked my kids." "Don't you think they deserve a spanking from time to time, like you did?" "Not at all. Physical violence is not my thing," he says solemnly. Even when some policemen use physical violence, their feelings about it are quite different from their parents'. Luis slapped his six-year-old daughter once, "but I cried after I did it. I felt so bad that I don't want to do it ever again."

Second, most of these men have probably chosen this occupation because it is closest to the notion of "educating through punishment." They not only enjoy punishing those who succumb to their base desires, but they also resolve their own problems—as the gays and the locusts do through their activities—through violence. In other words, the men who enforce the law seek to reenact the abuse for two purposes: in the first place, to "teach" others what they were taught as children through punishment; and second, to do so in a different way. By replacing the modality of excessive violence with a more moderate approach, the policemen try to tell themselves that there is no need to inflict the physical blows that they received as children.

HOMOPHOBIA

Policemen do not like gay men. The in-depth interviews reveal a great deal of hostility. Most of them perceive homosexuality as a vice indulged in by people who have strayed from the straight and narrow path. A minority believe that it is inherited as a result of hormonal disorders, and that those who suffer from this condition can do little to change it. This group is somewhat more tolerant toward gays. "They're ill," says Officer Pérez. "There's nothing you can do about it. We should feel sorry for them." However, this view is the exception. For most policemen, homosexuals are perverts who have chosen to embark on a life of crime, the same way that burglars have learned to steal. "Nobody is born with an inclination to steal," says Sergeant Fernández. "The same is true of drugs or homosexuality. If you take the wrong path, that's where you end up."

The police officers' homophobia is expressed in more subtle ways. When we asked whether they behaved differently toward gay men, since they considered homosexuality to be a crime, the answer was no. "Just because they are that way doesn't mean we discriminate against them," said Aron. Luis believes that every citizen deserves the same respect, "even if he is a criminal." However, the officers' actions suggest that discrimination is rampant.

One way of establishing differences in public places has to do with the sexual orientation of the couple. Police officers admit to being more tolerant of heterosexuals when they find them engaging in sexual activities in a public place. This tolerance is expressed in two ways: they are far less likely to arrest a heterosexual couple, and, as Sergeant Fernández says, they are more inclined to "let them finish what they're doing before intervening." When a police officer finds a heterosexual couple having sex, "one waits for them to finish before reprimanding them," says Roberto, another policeman.

Only one interviewee mentioned that a heterosexual couple had been arrested for having sex in a public place. Officer Chavez admitted that he had arrested the couple, both minors, "because I was just starting off and I didn't have much experience." He found a sixteen-year-old boy having sex with a fourteen-year-old girl. Chavez arrested them both, took them to the police station, and then he called their parents. "My boss chewed me out. 'Why did you get us into this?' he said. The girl's parents are going to break her when they find out.'" Nevertheless, Chavez told the parents what he had seen. "They just started kicking the girl, and they took her to a doctor to find out if she had lost her virginity."

When it comes to gay couples, police officers do not show such consideration. Policemen readily admit that when they run across two men having sex they feel that it is "revolting" (Aron), "repug-nant" (Chavez), or that it "makes me feel like vomiting" (Carlos). Officer Gutierrez feels "anger" while Ortega feels "nausea." Intervention is immediate and there is no question of waiting for the act to be consummated. In many cases, arrests are inevitable and in some violence plays a role. Luis admits that he will hit offenders with his baton a few times so they will learn "not to do such dirty things." Perez reprimands them "forcefully" for being so "revolting." Ortega tells them angrily to "get out of my sight." Fernandez pulls his gun on them "to scare them."

For the average policeman, gay men are people who belong to a higher social class but have not been properly raised. Too much luxury is what has led them to lose their discipline and moral fiber. If gays were poor, as policemen are, "they'd realize that life's not a party where you can get away with anything," says Fernandez. "Homosexuals weren't raised the way I was, and they allowed themselves to be led astray by vice and drugs," says Mario. For Perez, homosexuality is "pure shamelessness"; in other words, gays have no sense of decency or fear of God.

Policemen, therefore, see themselves as responsible for the "reeducation" of gay men. Most of them spend a fair amount of time telling them that "what they are doing is filthy," in Gutierrez's words. "They should learn that sex is only between men and women. Being a faggot is a waste," says Aron. All arrests or raids contain an element of "reeducation," of instilling "good citizen values."

It is possible that the police officers are re-enacting the abuse they were subjected to as children, in order to "educate" gay men, that is, to teach them how to control their own desires. In other words, they wish to discipline the gays as they were disciplined: through corporal punishment. It is hardly surprising, then, that some policemen should take this "discipline" to the same levels of abuse that they suffered. Many of our gay interviewees said they had suffered great violence at the hands of the police: beatings, torture, intimidation, and even rape. The same applies to the locusts. They are perceived by the police as beings dominated by improper material desires, who should learn to live like the police, with their aspirations firmly under control. "Criminals are people who haven't learned to control their vice, which is a lust for money . . . as if you can simply steal anything you want," says Officer Madrigal.

Although the cases above are true, we do not believe they are representative of most policemen's behavior. The gay men and locusts we interviewed admit that not all officers are violent toward them; many of them will preach rather than hit. Others ask them to leave the public place where they happen to be "so you don't get into trouble," and some even turn a blind eye when they realize that a couple are having sex. When asked what situations merited a violent response, gay sex in public places was not mentioned. It would appear that policemen's homophobia follows the same disciplinary model they learned at home: the body is punished to train it to behave "correctly." Some excesses may occur, but the ultimate goal is not violence, but "discipline."

IF YOU LIVE WITH MEN . . .

When asked about the reasons for muggings in public places, police officers who are not afraid of being politically incorrect blamed the gays. Miguel, one of the least homophobic officers interviewed, admits that when they get a call to investigate a mugging "my buddies go reluctantly, because they feel it was the queers who brought it upon themselves by deciding to fuck in those places." Sergeant Sanchez agrees. "What the hell is a momma's boy doing in a park at three in the morning? Isn't it crazy that we should have to go there to get him out of a mess?" Such attitudes suggest that the police would rather not intervene in the struggle between gays and locusts, and when they do their sympathies are with neither group.

However, there is a strong police presence in public places. The police do not let a day go by without patrolling these areas. Although crime levels are high throughout the country and people complain about the lack of officers patrolling the streets, the authorities make it a point to visit public parks during their rounds. When Fernández was asked why the police pay so much attention to La Llanura Park, and even have special mounted police units patrolling the area, he said:

> Look, the truth is we do it for the kids. Children are a country's greatest hope. Parks should be places where they can play with their families. How can we let them see a homosexual scene in a place like that? How low have we sunk when a little girl playing with her doll ends up seeing two men sucking each other's penises? How can we possibly not intervene to get rid of such filth in recreation areas?

Fernández's argument seemed reasonable enough. However, we were puzzled and asked, "What would a little girl be doing playing with her doll in a park at three in the morning?" "Don't be naive!" was the response. "Minors visit the park to prostitute themselves and smoke crack!" he said with a self-righteous air. "Yes, but then they're not kids who will be perverted by gays. Their heterosexual parents have already done that," we reply. "I agree," he said reluctantly. "But still, do you think it's good for a girl prostitute to see two guys kissing each other?"

Fernández's zeal in eradicating sex from public places is shared by the security guards at the University of the Republic campus. According to Officer Muñoz:

> To put a stop to all this filth, you always need to be vigilant. At night, I climb onto the rooftop of the highest building and I take my binoculars. From there I can see any strange activity that's going on, paying special attention to male couples. When I see one that's very close together, I climb down quickly and follow them. One night a couple went down to a little stream that flows through the campus and went under the bridge. To catch them, I had to crawl on my hands and knees so I wouldn't make any noise with my boots. Then I had to wait 'til they began having sex. Once their pants were down, I turned on the flashlight and arrested them.

Ernesto, a low-ranking policeman, has had considerable experience in preventing sex in movie theaters.

> I sit in the back row at the movies and keep my coat on so people can't tell I'm a policeman. Since they seem to find me attractive, there's usually some guy who will sit next to me. I

> pretend I'm watching the movie, but I'm all ears. The guy will stare at me a few times and I'll look at him just once, to pretend I'm interested. When the asshole touches my penis, I get up and go to the toilet. He follows me, thinking I'm into it. I get to the toilet and go into one of the cubicles and sit down on the toilet, leaving the door ajar. When the guy gets in, that's when I arrest him.

One possible explanation for this great zeal has to do with the very nature of the police corps. They are men who live, eat, work, play, and fight among men. Their bunks are next to one another; they use the same showers. Interaction is so intimate that they even have a saying to describe how they live: "At the police station, you hang your balls up at the door." This means that aggressive masculinity must be checked and that collective life in the station is "feminine," or intimate, even loving. If one leaves one's "balls" hanging on the door, one loses one's privileges as a male, and might even fall into the temptation of imitating the gay men who, in Sergeant Chavez's words, "walk around without their balls on." Hence the need to control the potential for homosexuality within the police corps. One way of doing it is to punish homosexuals, so that policemen can learn the price of giving free rein to their desires.

> Once they took me to a queers' bar without telling me. The captain said I should go out on patrol with my buddies. When we went inside, I saw mostly men and only a few women. However, I thought everything was normal and did not pay any attention. Suddenly I noticed that the men were dancing together and some were kissing each other. It was disgusting! I felt a horrible pain in my stomach and went to the bathroom to vomit. When I came out, my partners had all the customers lined up against the wall and were asking for their ID cards. I don't know why they didn't tell me we were going to a homosexual bar. What was the point of scaring me like that?

The "scare" is another lesson for the body: if you live intimately with other men, you should learn what happens to those who are tempted to love them.

DELIVER US FROM TEMPTATION

In spite of their best efforts to repress latent homosexuality in many policemen, or to control those who are already gay, the various police forces are only partially successful in their objective. Homosexual acts are not uncommon among policemen, and they are influenced by public sex. This is evident in many ways: voyeurism, participation, and even prostitution or bribe taking. Policemen, then, are another group that participates directly in public sex.

As we have seen, most policemen were trained to control their desires. However, when they come across gays and locusts, they see the faces of those who follow their urges. Both homosexuals and locusts struggle for the things that their bodies desire: sex and money. For instance, locusts mug people and steal things to buy drugs that will give pleasure to their bodies.

The first step toward participation in public sex is voyeurism. Policemen gradually become seduced by the sexual scenes they witness. Ernesto admits that he learned to let heterosexual couples "finish what they were doing." However, it was only later in the interview that he admitted to searching for them "more often than I'm ordered to." In other words, he learned to enjoy watching a couple having sex. Mario feels the same way. Even on his day off he will often go to porn movies to watch couples getting it on. "The more experience you have, the better you can do your job," is his excuse. Officer Morales is particularly fond of catching transvestites in parks. "I don't like homosexual sex, but when it's a transvestite with a man, I can't deny that I hang around a while to see how they do it. If a man is dressed up as a woman, it doesn't seem so repugnant," he says.

The next stage is to invite their spouses, girlfriends, or pickups to visit such places. Says Sargeant Pérez:

> After seeing so much filth in La Llanura, you begin to get kind of horny. Three months ago I met a girl who worked at a nearby store. We agreed to meet at the park. It was at night. There were lots of homosexual couples around. You can recognize them because they park their cars and start looking around for a pickup. My partner was very shy, but she said she liked policemen a lot. "Why, honey?" I asked her. "Is it be-

> cause you think we're rough?" "No," she said, "it's because you're so masculine and daring." Since she had given her consent, up to a point, I gave her a long kiss right there and then, in front of all the [gay] couples. A lot of queers were walking around, and they would stop to stare at us. But I wanted to show them how to do things properly. In the end, the woman allowed me to touch her all over, and I told her to sit down on the grass. When some guys came closer, I took out my penis and stuck it into her, lifting her skirt. It was a little uncomfortable, because I'd never done it in a public place before, and because the guys were masturbating while they were watching us.

Gregorio has also learned to enjoy the darkness of public parks. Over the past few months, he has been visiting Colombia Park as a place to have sex. When he is off-duty, he arranges to meet his girlfriends there and he claims he does things he would never have imagined.

> I've been getting bolder every day. It would never have occurred to me to have sex in the park. In fact, for several months, my job has been to put an end to it. However, for some time now I have found it a real turn-on. Last week I took this girl to the park. She was scared because she'd never done it [in such a place]. I told her not to worry, that I was a policeman and nothing could happen to us. The more frightened she looked when I touched her, the more turned on I was taking off her clothes. To make a long story short, I left her completely naked. I just put my coat over her.

A third step, which not everyone takes, is to participate in homosexual sex and sexual commerce. None of the policemen interviewed admitted to having done it, but they said that some of their colleagues had. Locusts and gays insist that many policemen force them to have sex with them, and then demand a bribe to let them go. This is what Jaime, a locust, had to say:

> I was with a client and two policemen showed up. They hit me with their baton and said, "You fucking queen, if you like

> sucking dick, you'd better suck ours, or we'll book you." Not only that—they also stole all my money.

José Julio, a sex worker, claims that policemen frequently steal the money he has earned and some have even raped him in the "cage" (the closed police van used to transport suspects to the police station):

> They told me I was under arrest for indecent behavior. They pushed me into the cage and drove around for about an hour. Then they stopped, and three cops got into the back, gagged me, and raped me.

Juan, a corporal, estimates that a policeman who accepts "gifts"—his name for bribes—can easily make up to two million colones (about $8,000) a month in public places. "That's a great temptation for people who don't have any money and who've had all kinds of limitations in their lives. Who gives a damn if someone is jacking off in a park at three in the morning?"

There is no such thing as an observer who is not influenced by the culture being observed.

Conclusion

In a Latin American country where the Catholic Church has banned sexual education, and family planning is accessible only to those who have managed to liberate themselves from religious dogma (the middle and upper classes of society), the poor continue to have more children than they can support. To be surrounded by children in an increasingly competitive economy, in which prices are constantly rising while job opportunities remain limited, provokes an accumulation of stress that people vent against their offspring. As we noted, nearly half of Costa Rica's children are either unwanted or unplanned, something that is borne out by the levels of child abuse in the families of our interviewees. It is hardly surprising, then, that many of them seek other avenues to "resolve" or "overcome" the abuse suffered previously, in public places. But it is not only the poor who are affected by the church's antisex stance. Homosexuals—a minority who are sufficiently weak not to pose a threat—are the prime target of attacks on immorality. Instead of focusing on infidelity and heterosexual promiscuity, the clergy specialize in promoting homophobia. In this way, they try to make us understand that they are fighting for Christian morals, despite the fact that the Church ignores the excesses of the majority of the population. Thus, the gays also experience great violence in a homophobic society, which they try to resolve as adults.

The disintegration of poor families because of their large size and the movement of the economy into a global marketplace has filled the country with criminals and *chapulines*. AIDS has also filled the country with gays who object to the way in which they have been treated, and are aware that traditional religious morality has allowed them to die like animals. At some imprecise moment in the past few years, these two groups began a small revolution in their repressed bodies. Without having planned it, and without even realizing what they were doing, they took over the public places of this small country to protest against the sexual and social repression experienced by minorities. What appears only as a source of pleasure cannot be separated from politics. For two men to dare to have oral sex in a park, something more than desire is required: an awareness that traditional morality and the prevailing sexual discourses do not include them. This break with traditional discourses that gays and *chapulines* enact every day in public places is a message for their friends and for everyone who pays attention. It might be expressed in a physical or nonverbal manner (after all, the poor and minorities have a particular problem with language that excludes them), but is it sufficiently clear for others, such as police officers, to have understood it? Or do we think that the police officer who chooses to have public sex is not trying to whisper something in our ear?

But the social protest which public sex represents cannot be seen simply as a cry of freedom. In some terrible way, it also repeats the oppression of the poor and the dispossessed. The locust who must sell his penis in a public park is not doing anything different than what his father did when he washed the car windshields of the middle classes. Once again, he is at the service of those who have the money to buy him. He is also ready to be abandoned when a better car washer or a bigger penis appears. The large number of gay men murdered by those who frequent public sex places is another kind of language. The locusts are saying something through these monstrous crimes. Real freedom from oppression cannot exist while some continue to dictate the discourses.

However, I do not wish to end this book on such a somber note. Perhaps we have made a great mistake by placing greater emphasis on violence than on the cordial relations that also exist among those who participate in public sex. We have mentioned that the majority of transactions take place without violence and that disputes and crimes are in a small minority. In this book we do not study many of the positive aspects of these transactions. Nevertheless, in these places many gays appear to acquire new skills in sexual communication and a greater appreciation of the potential of their sexual orientation. The mere fact of taking possession of a public place and making homosexuality visible in a society that had condemned gays to the closet is an act of bravery. Moreover, they have changed the traditional way in which homosexual desire and practice were expressed. This shows us that sexual orientation is not an unalterable construct, but is rather negotiated afresh every day, and makes Costa Rica's gay community one of the few who have succeeded in making changes to halt the advance of the AIDS epidemic.

The locusts also learn a great deal from the gays. They have learned that oppression is not a permanent state and have seen the gays defend their rights. In fact, the gays were the ones who took their protests to the country's Constitutional Court and succeeded in convincing it to ban indiscriminate raids and arbitrary arrests. This has directly benefitted the locusts and other groups who live or work on the streets.

Appendix

Survey of Sexual Practices in Public Sex Places

ILPES QUESTIONNAIRE FOR MEN WHO VISIT BARS, DISCOS, AND RESTAURANTS

We are carrying out a very important survey about sexual behavior. We are interviewing many people and we would like to ask for your cooperation. All the information you may provide will be strictly confidential. Your participation is voluntary, and you do not have to reply to any questions you do not wish to answer. May I begin the interview?

Activity	Name	Date	FOR OFFICE USE
Checked			A1. QUESTIONNAIRE #: /_/_/_/
Keyed in			
Verified			

A4.	NUMBER ON THE CONTROL SHEET	CODE /_/_/
A6.	PLACE WHERE THE INTERVIEW OCCURRED	CODE /_/_/
A8.	DATE OF THE INTERVIEW	DAY /_/_/ MONTH /_/_/
A12.	INTERVIEWER	CODE /_/_/
A14.	RESULTS OF THE INTERVIEW	RESULT /_/
A15.	TIME THE INTERVIEW BEGAN	HOUR /_/_/ MIN. /_/_/
A19.	To begin with, would you mind telling me how old you are?	AGE /_/_/
A21.	What was the highest grade you attained in formal education?	0. NONE 0 1. PRIMARY 1 2 3 4 5 6 2. SECONDARY 1 2 3 4 5+ 3. UNIVERSITY 1 2 3 4 5+

A23. What is your current marital status?	1. SINGLE 2. COMMON-LAW MARRIAGE 3. MARRIED 4. SEPARATED 5. DIVORCED 6. WIDOWER
A24. Do you currently live in the metropolitan area or outside of it?	1. METROPOLITAN AREA 2. OUTSIDE
A25. How would you define yourself in terms of your sexual orientation? **INTERVIEWER: PLEASE NOTE THE TERM USED BY THE INTERVIEWEE IN DESCRIBING HIMSELF SEXUALLY AND USE IT WHENEVER YOU RUN ACROSS THE FOLLOWING BRACKETS: [ ]**	1. HOMOSEXUAL/GAY 2. BISEXUAL 3. HETEROSEXUAL 4. TRANSVESTITE 5. TRANSSEXUAL (A WOMAN IN A MAN'S BODY) 6. *CACHERO* 7. OTHER: ____________ 8. DID NOT REPLY

I am going to mention a series of people or groups, so that you can tell me which of them know you are **[ ]**.	**DOES NOT HAVE ONE**	**YES**	**NO**	**WILL NOT SAY**	**Specify the % if there were several**
A26. Your closest heterosexual male friend?	1	2	3	4	▮▮▮▮▮▮▮▮▮▮
A27. Your closest heterosexual female friend?	1	2	3	4	▮▮▮▮▮▮▮▮▮▮
A28. Your immediate superior?	1	2	3	4	▮▮▮▮▮▮▮▮▮▮
A29. Your father?	1	2	3	4	▮▮▮▮▮▮▮▮▮▮
A30. Your mother?	1	2	3	4	▮▮▮▮▮▮▮▮▮▮
A31. Your brother(s)?	1	2	3	4	/_/_/_/%
A35. Your sister(s)?	1	2	3	4	/_/_/_/%
A39. Your wife?	1	2	3	4	▮▮▮▮▮▮▮▮▮▮
A40. Your child(ren)?	1	2	3	4	/_/_/_/%

A44. Now, speaking about your family, friends, and acquaintances, what percentage would you say *DO NOT KNOW* that you are **[ ]**, whether you have told them or not?	PERCENTAGE /_/_/_/%

<table>
<tr><td>A47. How old were you when you had your first sexual experience with a man?</td><td>AGE /_/_/
(WRITE DOWN "00" IF THE INTERVIEWEE CANNOT REMEMBER)</td></tr>
<tr><td>A49. Approximately how old was the person with whom you had your first sexual experience?</td><td>AGE /_/_/
(WRITE DOWN "00" IF THE INTERVIEWEE CANNOT REMEMBER)</td></tr>
<tr><td>A51. How was that person related to you?</td><td>01. FATHER
02. UNCLE
03. GRANDFATHER
04. BROTHER
05. COUSIN
06. FRIEND OF THE FAMILY
07. PERSONAL FRIEND
08. SCHOOLMATE
09. STRANGER
10. OTHER</td></tr>
</table>

A53. In terms of your general sexual activity, do you currently have sex with men, with women, or with women and men?

INTERVIEWER: PROBE AND DETERMINE WHICH OF THE FOLLOWING OPTIONS IS THE CORRECT ONE.

1. ONLY HAS SEX WITH MEN.
2. HAS SEX MAINLY WITH MEN, BUT OCCASIONALLY WITH WOMEN.
3. HAS SEX WITH BOTH MEN AND WOMEN.
4. HAS SEX MAINLY WITH WOMEN, BUT OCCASIONALLY WITH MEN.
5. ONLY HAS SEX WITH WOMEN.
6. DOES NOT HAVE SEX WITH EITHER MEN OR WOMEN.

A54. **INTERVIEWER: FOR THE FOLLOWING QUESTION, PLEASE HAND OUT CARD "A."**

Analyzing your current sexual partners, could you tell us, from your point of view, which of the following options best describes your current relationship?

1. CLOSED (A SINGLE REGULAR SEXUAL PARTNER).
2. OPEN (AT LEAST ONE REGULAR SEXUAL PARTNER, AND OTHER PARTNERS WHO MAY BE REGULAR OR OCCASIONAL).
3. DO NOT HAVE A REGULAR PARTNER, BUT DO HAVE OTHER OCCASIONAL PARTNERS.
4. CELIBATE WITH MEN (DOES NOT CURRENTLY HAVE SEX WITH MEN).
5. CELIBATE WITH WOMEN (DOES NOT CURRENTLY HAVE SEX WITH WOMEN).
6. OTHER: ______________________________

<table>
<tr><td>A55. Over the past twelve months, how many steady partners/lovers/companions have you had?</td><td>/_/_/_/_/
IF THE ANSWER IS "0000," PLEASE MOVE ON TO QUESTION A63.</td></tr>
<tr><td colspan="2">INTERVIEWER: IF NECESSARY, PLEASE TELL THE INTERVIEWEE THE FOLLOWING: "In our survey, we define as a steady partner, lover, or companion the man you have had sexual relations with once or more often, with whom you have sexual relations regularly, or whom you plan to continue having sex with." FIND OUT IF THE INTERVIEWEE UNDERSTOOD THE DEFINITION, AND REPEAT IT IF NECESSARY.</td></tr>
<tr><td>A59. Where did you meet your most recent steady partner/lover/companion?</td><td>01. BAR
02. DISCO
03. RESTAURANT
04. SCHOOL
05. SAUNA
06. PARK
07. PUBLIC SWIMMING POOL
08. MOVIE THEATER
09. ALLEYWAY
10. ABROAD
11. OTHER: ____________</td></tr>
<tr><td>A61. What was the name of the place?
NAME: ______________________________</td><td>CODE: /_/_/</td></tr>
<tr><td>A63. Over the past twelve months, how many occasional/sporadic/casual partners have you had?</td><td># /_/_/_/_/
IF THE ANSWER IS "0000," PLEASE MOVE ON TO QUESTION A71.</td></tr>
<tr><td colspan="2">INTERVIEWER: IF NECESSARY, PLEASE TELL THE INTERVIEWEE THE FOLLOWING: "In our survey, we define as an occasional/sporadic/casual partner a man you have had sexual relations with once or more often, with or without any commitment to have a future sexual encounter." FIND OUT IF THE INTERVIEWEE UNDERSTOOD THE DEFINITION, AND REPEAT IT IF NECESSARY.</td></tr>
<tr><td>A67. Where did you meet your last occasional/sporadic/casual partner?</td><td>01. BAR
02. DISCO
03. RESTAURANT
04. SCHOOL
05. SAUNA
06. PARK
07. PUBLIC SWIMMING POOL
08. MOVIE THEATER
09. ALLEYWAY
10. ABROAD
11. OTHER: ____________</td></tr>
<tr><td>A69. What was the name of the place?
NAME: ______________________________</td><td>CODE: /_/_/</td></tr>
</table>

A71. Over the past thirty days, how many different people have you had sex with?	PARTNERS: /_/_/_/_/ **IF THE ANSWER IS "0000," PLEASE MOVE ON TO QUESTION B4.**
A73. Over those same thirty days, did you have sex most of the time with your regular partner or with others?	1. PARTNER 2. OTHERS

Now I am going to ask you some very personal questions that are very important for our survey. Please help me by replying as accurately as possible.

How easy or difficult is it for you to ask these things of the person you are about to have a first sexual contact with?	**VERY EASY**	**EASY**	**REGU-LAR**	**DIFFI-CULT**	**VERY DIFFI-CULT**
B4. Asking him to have sex with you.	1	2	3	4	5
B5. Being asked to have sex with him.	1	2	3	4	5
B6. Saying to him that you want to perform oral sex on him without a condom.	1	2	3	4	5
B7. Saying to him that you want to perform oral sex on him with a condom.	1	2	3	4	5
B8. Asking him to perform oral sex on you without a condom.	1	2	3	4	5
B9. Asking him to perform oral sex on you with a condom.	1	2	3	4	5
B10. Asking him to come in your mouth.	1	2	3	4	5
B11. Asking him not to come in your mouth.	1	2	3	4	5
B12. Asking him if you can come in his mouth.	1	2	3	4	5
B13. Asking him if he can perform oral sex on you without you coming in his mouth.	1	2	3	4	5
B14. Asking him if you can penetrate him with a condom.	1	2	3	4	5
B15. Asking him if you can penetrate him without a condom.	1	2	3	4	5

B16. Asking him to penetrate you with a condom.	1	2	3	4	5
B17. Asking him to penetrate you without a condom.	1	2	3	4	5
B18. Saying that you want to ejaculate inside him.	1	2	3	4	5
B19. Asking him to ejaculate inside you.	1	2	3	4	5
B20. Asking him to penetrate you, but not to ejaculate inside you.	1	2	3	4	5
B21. Performing oral sex on your partner without a condom after he penetrated you.	1	2	3	4	5
B22. Performing oral sex on your partner with a condom after he penetrated you.	1	2	3	4	5
B23. Licking your partner's anus after having penetrated him.	1	2	3	4	5
B24. Licking your partner's nipples.	1	2	3	4	5
B25. Having your nipples licked.	1	2	3	4	5
B26. Being kissed on the mouth.	1	2	3	4	5
B27. Not being kissed on the mouth.	1	2	3	4	5
B28. Asking your partner if he has a venereal disease.	1	2	3	4	5
B29. Asking your partner if he has HIV/AIDS.	1	2	3	4	5
B30. Telling your partner that a part of his body smells.	1	2	3	4	5
B31. Asking your partner to bathe before having sex.	1	2	3	4	5
B32. Telling your partner he smells.	1	2	3	4	5
B33. Asking your partner to wash his penis if it smells.	1	2	3	4	5
B34. Telling your partner that you want to use sex toys.	1	2	3	4	5

B35. Telling your partner that you do not want to use sex toys.	1	2	3	4	5
How repugnant do you find the following bodily fluids and solids?	**VERY REPUG-NANT**	**REPUG-NANT**	**MORE OR LESS REPUG-NANT**	**SOME-WHAT REPUG-NANT**	**NOT AT ALL REPUG-NANT**
B36. Tears	1	2	3	4	5
B37. Sweat	1	2	3	4	5
B38. Saliva	1	2	3	4	5
B39. Semen	1	2	3	4	5
B40. Blood	1	2	3	4	5
B41. Urine	1	2	3	4	5
B42. Feces (shit)	1	2	3	4	5

Please answer "yes" or "no" to the following statements.	**YES**	**NO**
B43. Have you ever been beaten when you were having sex?	1	2
B44. Have you ever beaten someone with whom you were having sex?	1	2
B45. Have you ever been immobilized while you were having sex?	1	2
B46. Have you ever immobilized your partner while you were having sex?	1	2
B47. Have you ever insulted your partner while you were having sex?	1	2
B48. Have you ever been insulted by your partner while you were having sex?	1	2
B49. Have you ever been physically forced to have sex?	1	2
B50. Have you ever physically forced someone to have sex?	1	2
B51. Have you ever played violent games while having sex?	1	2

B52. Please say if you agree or disagree with the following statement: The sensation of danger or risk makes sex more exciting.	1. AGREE 2. DISAGREE 3. NOT SURE

B53. How frequently do you feel an uncontrollable urge to have sex?	1. ALWAYS 2. NEARLY ALWAYS 3. SOMETIMES 4. HARDLY EVER 5. NEVER **(PLEASE GO ON TO QUESTION B61.)**
B54. How frequently do you satisfy this urge?	1. ALWAYS 2. NEARLY ALWAYS 3. SOMETIMES 4. HARDLY EVER 5. NEVER **(PLEASE GO ON TO QUESTION B61.)**

How do you satisfy this urge?	**SPONTA-NEOUS**	**WITH PROMPTING**	
	YES	**YES**	**NO**
B55. You masturbate.	1	2	3
B56. You have sex with your steady partner.	1	2	3
B57. You have sex with someone you know.	1	2	3
B58. You have sex with someone you do not know.	1	2	3
B59. You engage in group sex.	1	2	3
B60. Other: ______________________	1	2	3

I will now give you a card that includes the names of ten places, and I would like you to rate them from 1 to 10 according to how erotic you feel they are as a place to have sex. Number 1 stands for the most erotic place, number 10 for the least erotic.
(INTERVIEWER: PLEASE HAND OVER CARD "B")

B61. An alleyway	01	02	03	04	05	06	07	08	09	10
B63. A movie theater	01	02	03	04	05	06	07	08	09	10
B65. The countryside	01	02	03	04	05	06	07	08	09	10
B67. A house	01	02	03	04	05	06	07	08	09	10
B69. An apartment	01	02	03	04	05	06	07	08	09	10
B71. A motel	01	02	03	04	05	06	07	08	09	10
B73. A public toilet	01	02	03	04	05	06	07	08	09	10
B75. An urban park	01	02	03	04	05	06	07	08	09	10
B77. A sauna	01	02	03	04	05	06	07	08	09	10
B79. A vehicle	01	02	03	04	05	06	07	08	09	10

Now I am going to mention several places, and I would like you to tell me if you have visited any of them to have sex.	YES	NO
C4. La Sabana Metropolitan Park	1	2
C5. National Park	1	2
C6. Central Park	1	2
C7. University of Costa Rica Campus	1	2
C8. Ojo de Agua Spa	1	2
C9. Alleyway	1	2
C10. Sauna	1	2
C11. Movie theater	1	2
C12. Public toilet	1	2
C13. Other 1: ____________________	1	2
C14. Other 2: ____________________	1	2
C15. Other 3: ____________________	1	2

INTERVIEWER: PLEASE INDICATE WHETHER THE INTERVIEWEE REPLIED AFFIRMATIVELY TO ANY OF THE ABOVE OPTIONS. IF SO, ASK THE FOLLOWING QUESTIONS. IF NOT, MOVE ON TO QUESTION C59.
1. YES
2. NO **(MOVE ON TO QUESTION C59.)**

Which of the following situations prompt you to visit such places?	YES	NO
C17. Having sex without a feeling of commitment.	1	2
C18. Having sex with strangers.	1	2
C19. Having a quickie.	1	2
C20. "Scoring" for sex quickly.	1	2
C21. Having sex without the need to engage in conversation.	1	2
C22. Doing something you consider taboo.	1	2
C23. Enjoying the thrill of knowing you might be found out.	1	2
C24. Enjoying the feeling of risk attached to such a place.	1	2
C25. Not wanting to be identified as a homosexual.	1	2
C26. Having sex with several people at the same time.	1	2
C27. Feeling unattractive.	1	2
C28. Having trouble picking people up for sex in bars or discos.	1	2
C29. Getting some money.	1	2
C30. Being able to afford to pay someone to have sex with you.	1	2

C31. Feeling lonely.	1	2
C32. Having sex with aggressive people.	1	2
C33. Experiencing the constant need to meet new people.	1	2
C34. Having drunk alcohol.	1	2
C35. Having taken drugs.	1	2
C36. Having sex mostly in such places.	1	2
C37. Enjoying the sight of other people having sex.	1	2
C38. Enjoying other people watching you having sex with someone.	1	2
C39. Having sex with different people all the time.	1	2
C40. Other: ______________________	1	2

C41. Who goes with you to those places?	1. NO ONE 2. FRIEND(S) 3. MY PARTNER 4. OTHER: __________
C42. How frequently do you visit those places?	1. MORE THAN TWICE A WEEK 2. ONCE A WEEK 3. ONCE A MONTH 4. A FEW TIMES A YEAR

Specifically, which of the following activities do you engage in there?	**SPONTANEOUS**	**WITH PROMPTING**	
	YES	**YES**	**NO**
C43. Watching.	1	2	3
C44. Making friends.	1	2	3
C45. Masturbating someone.	1	2	3
C46. Having someone masturbate you.	1	2	3
C47. Performing oral sex on someone.	1	2	3
C48. Having someone perform oral sex on you.	1	2	3
C49. Penetrating someone.	1	2	3
C50. Being penetrated by someone.	1	2	3
C51. Going off with someone to his home.	1	2	3
C52. Taking someone home with you.	1	2	3
C53. Other: ______________________	1	2	3

C54. The last time you had sex in any of these places, did you engage in penetration?	1. YES 2. NO **(PLEASE MOVE ON TO QUESTION C57.)**
C55. Did someone use a condom?	1. YES 2. NO **(PLEASE MOVE ON TO QUESTION C57.)**
C56. Who used it?	1. THE INTERVIEWEE 2. HIS SEXUAL PARTNER 3. BOTH
C57. The last time you visited one of these places, did you drink alcohol?	1. YES 2. NO
C58. Did you take drugs?	1. YES 2. NO
C59. Changing the subject, do you have a closer relationship with your mother's or your father's side of the family?	1. MOTHER'S SIDE 2. FATHER'S SIDE 3. BOTH 4. NEITHER
C60. How many of your uncles and cousins on your mother's side of the family do you know are gay?	# /_/_/ **(WRITE DOWN "00" IF THE ANSWER IS "I DON'T KNOW.")**
C62. How many of your aunts and female cousins on your mother's side of the family do you know are lesbians?	# /_/_/ **(WRITE DOWN "00" IF THE ANSWER IS "I DON'T KNOW.")**
C64. How many of your uncles and cousins on your father's side of the family do you know are gay?	# /_/_/ **(WRITE DOWN "00" IF THE ANSWER IS "I DON'T KNOW.")**
C66. How many of your aunts and female cousins on your father's side of the family do you know are lesbians?	# /_/_/ **(WRITE DOWN "00" IF THE ANSWER IS "I DON'T KNOW.")**

Do you recall being the victim of some kind of severe emotional abuse, such as insults, yelling, being ridiculed, being rejected or criticized, etc.?	**YES**	**NO**	**CAN-NOT RECALL**	**N/A**
C68. Before you were 12?	1	2	3	▮▮▮▮▮▮▮▮
C69. Between the ages of 12 and 18?	1	2	3	▮▮▮▮▮▮▮▮
C70. Currently, by your partner?	1	2	▮▮▮▮▮▮▮▮	8
C71. Currently, by other people?	1	2	▮▮▮▮▮▮▮▮	▮▮▮▮▮▮▮▮

Do you recall being the victim of some kind of intense physical abuse, such as being pinched, slapped, punched, kicked, being hit in different parts of the body, suffering fractures, etc.?	YES	NO	CAN-NOT RECALL	N/A
C72. Before you were 12?	1	2	3	
C73. Between the ages of 12 and 18?	1	2	3	
C74. Currently, by your partner?	1	2		8
C75. Currently, by other people?	1	2		
C76. Do you recall being forced to engage in acts of a sexual nature?				
C77. Before you were twelve?	1	2	3	
C78. Between the ages of 12 and 18?	1	2	3	
C79. Currently, by your partner?	1	2		8
C80. Currently, by other people?	1	2		

D4. Changing the subject, how handsome do you consider yourself to be?	1. VERY HANDSOME 2. HANDSOME 3. AVERAGE 4. NOT VERY HANDSOME 5. NOT HANDSOME AT ALL
D5. How handsome do you believe others consider you to be?	1. VERY HANDSOME 2. HANDSOME 3. AVERAGE 4. NOT VERY HANDSOME 5. NOT HANDSOME AT ALL
D6. How easy is it for you to pick up someone?	1. EASY 2. AVERAGE 3. DIFFICULT
D7. Finally, how many days a month do you visit this place?	# DAYS /_/_/
D9. TIME THE INTERVIEW WAS CONCLUDED:	HOUR /_/_/ MIN. /_/_/

INTERVIEWER:
- **ASK THE INTERVIEWEE FOR AN EXTRA MINUTE TO GO OVER THE QUESTIONNAIRE AND VERIFY THAT IT WAS COMPLETED CORRECTLY.**
- **SAY THANK YOU AND FINISH THE INTERVIEW.**

D13. DEGREE OF COOPERATION	1. VERY GOOD 2. GOOD 3. AVERAGE 4. POOR 5. VERY POOR

D14. VALIDITY OF THE ANSWERS	1. VERY GOOD 2. GOOD 3. AVERAGE 4. POOR 5. VERY POOR
D15. OTHER PEOPLE PRESENT AT THE TIME OF THE INTERVIEW	1. NOBODY 2. PARTNER 3. FRIENDS 4. OTHERS

FOR OFFICE USE

D16. ESTABLISHMENT /_/

D17. UPM # /_/

D18. # OF THE TOTAL /_/_/

Notes

Introduction

1. Michel Foucault, *Histoire de la Sexualité. La Volonté de Savoir,* Vol. 1, Paris: Gallimard, 1976.
2. Michel Foucault, *The Birth of the Clinic.* Mexico: Siglo XXI, 1991.
3. *La Nación,* "Virgen en Talamanca," Viva supplement, April 18, 1998, p. 1.
4. Jacobo Schifter, *La Formación de una Contracultura: Homosexualismo y SIDA en Costa Rica* (The Development of a Counter Culture: Homosexuality and AIDS in Costa Rica), San José, Costa Rica: Guayacán, 1989.
5. Jacobo Schifter and Johnny Madrigal, *Las Gavetas Sexuales del Costarricense y el Riesgo de Infección con el VIH* (The Sexual Compartments of the Costa Rican and the Risk of HIV Infection), San José, Costa Rica: IMEDIEX, 1996, p. 5.
6. Victor Hugo Acuña, "Historia económica del tabaco en Costa Rica." ("Economic history of tobacco in Costa Rica.") *Anuario de Estudios Centroamericanos,* No. 4, 1978, pp. 20-40.
7. Ricardo Blanco, *Historia Eclesiástica de Costa Rica: Del Descubrimiento a la Erección de la Diócesis (1502-1850)* (Ecclesiastical History of Costa Rica: From the Discovery to the Establishment of the Diocese [1502-1850]), San José, Costa Rica: Editorial, 1994.
8. Jacobo Schifter and Johnny Madrigal, *Las Gavetas Sexuales del Costarricense y el Riesgo de Infección con el VIH,* p. 5.
9. Jeannette Cover, "Abuso Sexual Infantil en Poblaciones Universitarias" (Childhood Sexual Abuse in University Populations). Thesis for postgraduate degree in psychology University of Costa Rica 1995.
10. Isabel Brenes, "Actitudes y Prácticas del Aborto Inducido en Costa Rica" (Attitudes and Practice of Induced Abortion in Costa Rica.). Thesis for master's degree in statistics. University of Costa Rica, 1994.
11. Victor Gomez, *Encuesta Nacional de Salud Reproductiva: Fecundidad y Formación de la Familia* (National Reproductive Health Survey: Fertility and Family Education), San José, Costa Rica: Department of Preventive Medicine, Reproductive Health Program, CCSS, 1994.
12. Ibid.
13. Jacobo Schifter and Johnny Madrigal, *Hombres Que Aman Hombres* (Men Who Love Men), San José, Costa Rica: Editorial ILEP-SIDA, 1992, pp. 390-391.
14. Joseph Carrier, *De los Otros: Intimacy and Homosexuality Among Mexican Men,* New York: Columbia University Press, 1995, p. 7.

15. K.F. Wolff, *The Sociology of Georg Simmel,* London: Collier Macmillan, 1950.

16. John D'Emilio, *Sexual Politics, Sexual Communities: The Making of a Homosexual Minority in the United States, 1940-1970,* Chicago: The University of Chicago Press, 1983.

17. Jacobo Schifter and Johnny Madrigal, *Las Gavetas Sexuales del Costarricense y el Riesgo de Infección con el VIH,* p. 99.

18. Department for AIDS Control, Costa Rican Health Ministry. "AIDS report up to July 1998."

19. Jacobo Schifter, *La Formación de Una Contracultura: Homosexualismo y SIDA en Costa Rica,* pp. 272-273.

20. ILPES, Half-yearly and annual work reports, 1993-1998.

21. Jacobo Schifter and Johnny Madrigal, *Hombres Que Aman Hombres,* p. 447.

22. Gary W. Dowsett, *Practicing Desire: Homosexual Sex in the Era of AIDS,* Stanford, CA: Stanford University Press, 1996.

23. Ibid., p. 46.

24. Joseph Carrier, *De los Otros: Intimacy and Homosexuality Among Mexican Men.*

25. Antonio de Moya and Rafael Garcia, "Three decades of male sex work in Santo Domingo," in Peter Aggleton, ed., *Men Who Sell Sex,* London: UCL Press, 1998, pp. 127-139.

26. For the 1989 and 1998 surveys, a list of gay bars, saunas, movie theaters, and gay meeting places was drawn up. In response to requests by some of these, we decided not to include any names so as to protect their identity.

27. Jacobo Schifter and Johnny Madrigal, *Hombres Que Aman Hombres,* pp. 439-442.

28. Jacobo Schifter and Johnny Madrigal, *Las Gavetas Sexuales del Costarricense y el Riesgo de Infección con el VIH.*

29. Statistics from the Department for AIDS Control, Costa Rican Health Ministry, San José, Costa Rica, 1998.

Chapter 1

1. Jacobo Schifter and Johnny Madrigal, *Hombres Que Aman Hombres.* San José, Costa Rica: Editorial ILEP-SIDA, 1992.

2. Ibid.

3. Jacobo Schifter, *Lila's House: Male Prostitution in Latin America,* Binghamton, NY: The Haworth Press, Inc., 1998.

4. Joseph Carrier, *De los Otros: Intimacy and Homosexuality Among Mexican Men,* New York: Columbia University Press, 1995, p. 11.

5. E. Antonio de Moya and Rafael Garcia, "Three decades of male sex work in Santo Domingo," in Peter Aggleton, ed., *Men Who Sell Sex,* London: UCL Press, 1998, pp. 127-139.

6. Jacobo Schifter, *Macho Love: Sex Behind Bars in Central America,* Binghamton, NY: The Haworth Press, Inc., 1999.

7. N. Coombs, "Male prostitution: A psychological view of behavior," *American Journal of Orthopsychiatry*, 44 (5):782-789, 1974.

8. J. Jersild, *Boy Prostitution.* Copenhagen: C.E.C. Gad, 1956.

9. K. Ginsburg, "The meat rack: A study of the male homosexual prostitute." *American Journal of Psychotherapy*, 21 (2):170-185, 1967.

10. Rudi C. Bleys, *The Geography of Perversion: Male to Male Sexual Behavior Outside the West and the Ethnographic Imagination 1750-1918,* New York: New York University Press, 1995.

11. Jacobo Schifter and Johnny Madrigal, *Las Gavetas Sexuales del Costarricense y el Riesgo del Infección con el VIH,* San José, Costa Rica: Editorial IMEDIEX, 1996.

12. Jacobo Schifter, *Lila's House: Male Prostitution in Latin America.*

13. P. Gandy, "Environmental and Psychological Factors in the Origin of the Young Male Prostitute." Paper presented to the American Anthropological Association, November 20, 1970; P. Gandy and R. Deisher, "Young male prostitutes: The physician's role in social rehabilitation," *Journal of the American Medical Association*, 212 (10):1661-1666, 1970.

14. S. Raven, "Boys will be boys," *Encounter*, 86:19, 1960.

15. E. Antonio de Moya and Rafael Garcia, "Three decades of male sex work in Santo Domingo," in Peter Aggleton, ed., *Men Who Sell Sex,* London: UCL Press, 1998.

Chapter 2

1. He is referring to the 1856 invasion by William Walker, a southerner who invaded Nicaragua and then tried to conquer Costa Rica.

2. Jacobo Schifter and Johnny Madrigal, *Hombres Que Aman Hombres,* San José, Costa Rica: Editorial ILEP-SIDA, 1992, p. 381.

Chapter 4

1. Jacques Derrida, *Of Grammatology,* Baltimore: The Johns Hopkins University Press, 1976.

2. Laud Humphreys, *Tearoom Trade: Impersonal Sex in Public Places,* Second Edition. New York: Aldine de Gruyter, 1975, p. 108.

3. Matt Adams, *Hustlers, Escorts and Porn Stars: The Insider's Guide to Male Prostitution in America,* Las Vegas, NV, Adams, 1999, p. 62.

4. Professor at the University of Chicago and winner of the Nobel Prize for Economics.

5. Pat Califia, *Public Sex: The Culture of Radical Sex,* San Francisco: Cleis Press, 1994.

Chapter 5

1. Joseph Carrier, *De los Otros: Intimacy and Homosexuality Among Mexican Men,* New York: Columbia University Press, 1995, p. 45.

Chapter 6

1. Mike Lew, *Victims No Longer: Men Recovering from Incest and Other Sexual Child Abuse,* New York: HarperCollins, 1988.

Chapter 7

1. Emmanuel Levinas, *Outside the Subject.* London: The Athlone Press, 1993.
2. Louis A. Sass, *Madness and Modernism: Insanity in the Light of Modern Art, Literature, and Thought.* Cambridge/London: The Harvard University Press, 1994, p. 98.
3. Michel Foucault, *La Historia de la Sexualidad.* (The History of Sexuality), Volume 1, Mexico: Siglo XXI, 1991.
4. Ibid.
5. A *cachero* is a heterosexual man who engages in active sex with men and who is not considered a homosexual in Latin American culture. More information on this subject may be found in Jacobo Schifter, *Lila's House: Male Prostitution in Latin America,* Binghamton, NY: The Haworth Press, Inc., 1998.
6. *Chapulines* or locusts are street kids who operate in gangs robbing and mugging people in urban areas.
7. Alfredo Mirandé, *Hombres y Machos: Masculinity and Latin Culture,* Boulder, CO: Westview Press, 1997.
8. N. Coombs, "Male prostitution: A psychological view of behavior," *American Journal of Orthopsychiatry,* 44 (5):782-789, 1974.
9. El Salon is an AIDS prevention project launched by ILPES in 1997, for sex workers and delinquents. For reasons of confidentiality, no details of its location are given.
10. D. Russel, "From the Massachusetts court clinics: On the psychopathology of boy prostitutes," *International Journal of Offender Therapy,* 15:42-52, 1971.
11. D. MacNamara, "Male prostitution in American cities: A sociological or pathological phenomenon?" *American Journal of Orthopsychiatry,* 35:204, 1965.
12. Cudore L. Snell, *Young Men in the Street: Help-Seeking Behavior of Young Male Prostitutes,* Westport, CT: Praeger, 1995, p. 38.
13. Margaret Gibson, "Clitoral corruption, body metaphors, and American doctors: Construction of female sexuality, 1870-1900," in Vernon A. Rosario, ed., *Science and Homosexualities,* New York: Routledge, 1997, pp. 108-133.

Chapter 8

1. Martin Kantor, *Homophobia: Description, Development, and Dynamics of Gay Bashing,* Westport, CT: Praeger, 1998.
2. Ibid., p. 97.
3. These specific interviews were carried out by Antonio Bustamante.

4. Robert P. MacNamara, *The Times Square Hustler: Male Prostitution in New York City,* Westport, CT: Praeger, 1994.

5. Pat Califia, *Public Sex: The Culture of Radical Sex,* Pittsburgh, PA: Cleis Press, 1994.

Chapter 9

1. Translator's note: In Costa Rica, as in many other countries, police officers continue to be overwhelmingly male.

Index

Page numbers followed by the letter "t" indicate tables.

MORE PUBLISHED BOOKS FROM HAWORTH GAY & LESBIAN STUDIES

4 Scintillating books by Steven Zeeland!
Visit Steven Zeeland at his home page:
http://www.stevenzeeland.com

MILITARY TRADE

NEW!

Over 250 Pages!

#1 on The Advocate's Men's Titles Hot Sellers List, June 1999!

"Once again, Steve Zeeland has pulled off the masterful and the unpredictable. This book is a document of scholarly importance—to historians, to sociologists, to students of gender and masculinity, and the mores of modern military life—and it is a smoldering seductive passage into the labyrinths of man-sex that disturbs, intrigues, and arouses as you sit up all night trying to put it down."
—Frank Browning, Author, *The Culture of Desire* and *Queer Geography*

$49.95 hard. ISBN: 0-7890-0402-X.
$19.95 soft. ISBN: 1-56023-924-7.
1999. Available now. 266 pp. with Index.

THE MASCULINE MARINE

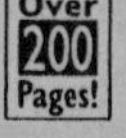

Homoeroticism in the U.S. Marine Corps

"A startlingly successful amalgam of contemporary gay theory about gender and the nature of manhood."
—*Manifest Reader*

This exciting book was listed as #1 on *The Advocate's* bestseller list for December 1996!

$39.95 hard. ISBN: 1-56024-982-X.
$14.95 soft. ISBN: 1-56023-874-7. 1996. 203 pp.

SAILORS AND SEXUAL IDENTITY

Over 250 Pages!

Crossing the Line Between "Straight" and "Gay" in the U.S. Navy

"May startle even those of us who have been the most suspicious of the 'straightness' of the Navy."
—*Cross-Talk*

The conversations in this book reveal how known "gay" and "straight" men can and do get along in the sexually tense confines of barracks and shipboard life once they discover that the imagined boundary between them is not, in fact, a hard line.

$39.95 hard. ISBN: 1-56024-850-5.
$14.95 soft. ISBN: 1-56023-850-X.
1995. 296 pp. Illustrations.

BARRACK BUDDIES AND SOLDIER LOVERS

Over 250 Pages!

Dialogues with Gay Young Men in the U.S. Military

"Describes an informal network of gay American GIs and civilians based in Frankfurt, Germany, shortly before the Gulf war."
—*Newsweek*

This book is a look around at current events in gay military circles from the eyes of these gay or bisexual military men, all of whom were stationed in Frankfurt, Germany, during the 1990s.

$39.95 hard. ISBN: 1-56024-377-5.
$14.95 soft. ISBN: 1-56023-032-0. 1993. 293 pp.

ACTS OF DISCLOSURE

The Coming-Out Process of Contemporary Gay Men
Marc E. Vargo, MS

"A singularly fair and even-handed evaluation of the pluses and minuses of coming out."
—*Michael's Thing*

$49.95 hard. ISBN: 0-7890-0236-1.
$17.95 soft. ISBN: 1-56023-912-3. 1998. 164 pp. with Index.
Features a list of coming-out resources, appendixes, and a bibliography.

THE EMPRESS IS A MAN

Over 200 Pages!

Stories from the Life of José Sarria
Michael R. Gorman, MA

"A biography of one of the most colorful and important figures of queer history since the second world war."
—*The Harvard Gay & Lesbian Review*

$39.95 hard. ISBN: 0-7890-0259-0.
$19.95 soft. ISBN: 1-56023-917-4. 1998. 278 pp. with Index.
Features photographs and interviews!

TWENTY MILLION NEW CUSTOMERS!

Over 200 Pages!

Understanding Gay Men's Consumer Behavior
Steven M. Kates, CA, MBA, PhD

"A fascinating exploration of the complicated role the market and consumption play in the gay male community."
—*Lambda Book Report*

$39.95 hard. ISBN: 0-7890-0175-6.
$19.95 soft. ISBN: 1-56023-903-4.
1997. 235 pp. with Index.
Features interviews and a bibliography.

FOUNDATIONS OF SOCIAL WORK PRACTICE WITH LESBIAN AND GAY PERSONS

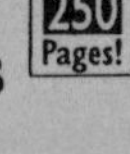

Edited by Gerald P. Mallon, DSW

Provides you with critical information that will help you in pursuing economic and social equality for diverse and at-risk client populations.

$49.95 hard. ISBN: 0-7890-0348-1.
$22.95 soft. ISBN: 1-56023-101-7.
1997. 298 pp. with Index.
Includes an Instructor's Manual.

INCLUDES INSTRUCTOR'S MANUAL FREE WITH DESK COPY!

AVAILABLE FROM YOUR LOCAL BOOKSTORE

If unavailable at your local bookstore, contact: Harrington Park Press,
10 Alice Street, Binghamton, New York 13904–1580 USA
Phone: 1–800–Haworth (Outside US/Canada + 607–722–5857)
Fax: 1–800–895–0582 (Outside US/Canada + 607–771–0012)
E-Mail: getinfo@haworthpressinc.com • Web: http://www.haworthpressinc.com

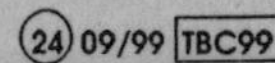